Dr Robert Youngson is a member of the
Royal College of Surgeons and Fellow of the
Royal Society of Medicine. He is also the
Army's Consultant Advisor in
Opthalmology.

He is the author of several self-help books
including *Everything You Need to Know
About Your Eyes* and *How to Cope with
Tinnitus and Hearing Loss*. He is currently
writing a book about strokes.

Learning to Live with Diabetes

Dr R.M. Youngson

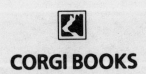

CORGI BOOKS

LEARNING TO LIVE WITH DIABETES

A CORGI BOOK 0 552 99263 1

First publication in Great Britain

PRINTING HISTORY
Corgi edition published 1987

This book is set in 11/12 pt Cheltenham
by Colset Private Limited, Singapore.

Corgi Books are published by Transworld Publishers Ltd.,
61–63 Uxbridge Road, Ealing, London W5 5SA, in Australia by
Transworld Publishers (Australia) Pty. Ltd., 15–23 Helles
Avenue, Moorebank, NSW 2170, and in New Zealand by
Transworld Publishers (N.Z.) Ltd., Cnr. Moselle and Waipareira
Avenues, Henderson, Auckland.

Made and printed in Great Britain by
The Guernsey Press Co. Ltd., Guernsey, Channel Islands.

Contents

PREFACE

So you're a diabetic?

Well, you're in good company. There are a million of you in Britain alone. Maybe you attend a diabetic clinic. Ideally you should, because that's where the experts are to be found and you deserve all the help you can get. But the chances are that, unless you are an adolescent, or a 'brittle' diabetic, or pregnant, you probably don't have this advantage. Regrettably, there are just too many diabetics and not enough clinics. So it has now become accepted that most adult diabetics must, at least to some extent, accept responsibility for their own day-to-day care. And that probably means you. It also means that, somehow, you have to get a firm understanding of the principles of diabetes and of its management. Education in this must be of central concern to you.

Your GP is well aware of the importance of this, but where is he to find the time to teach you? Doctors and nurses will certainly do what they can for you, but you are really going to have to do quite a lot for yourself. If you acknowledge this – if you are determined to have an intelligent grasp of diabetes and all its implications – then this book is dedicated to you.

Dr Robert Youngson, 1986.

1 WHAT IS DIABETES?

If you are a diabetic, one thing is quite essential – that you
should understand diabetes. This is basic to your future
health and happiness. Many people drive cars without
having the least idea of how the engine works, or enjoy TV
without knowing the first thing about electronics. But if you
are diabetic and neglect to master the principles of the subject, you do so at your peril. You can't just live with diabetes
and put up with it, as you might live with chronic bronchitis
or dyslexia. Diabetes is a condition you have to manage –
actively, sensibly and continuously – if you are going to
stay healthy. For a few diabetics, management is simple –
just a matter of watching the diet – but for most, the matter
is much more complicated and the consequences of neglect
much more serious.

OK, this is bad luck – very bad luck. Diabetes is a great
nuisance and quite a worry, too. Urine tests, insulin injections, hypoglycaemia, strict diet control. You may even feel
bitter and resentful that it should have happened to you. But
the fact is that you are stuck with it and resentment isn't
going to help. What will help is a positive, constructive attitude based on a clear understanding of what diabetes is all
about and a determination that you are going to beat the
disease, rather than let the disease beat you. And that is the
purpose of this book – to explain diabetes, to induce in you
an enlightened and optimistic attitude to the condition and
to show you how, in spite of your diabetes, to live a full and
unrestricted life.

Let me start by telling you a story. Read it carefully,
because it has much to tell you about diabetes.

What happened to Michael

Michael felt terribly tired. For weeks he had been less ener-
getic than normal and often just sat around doing nothing.
He knew he should be working for his 'O' levels but he just
didn't feel up to it. He had even lost interest in his computer.
And his clothes – they were so loose – just hanging on him.
It was strange, too, how thirsty he seemed to be. One glass
of orange squash was never enough and he was always
making himself great mugs of coffee. Of course, the result
was that he was never out of the toilet. He even had to get
up at night. And once he had splashed the leg of his blue
pyjamas and the urine had dried leaving a white stain.

One day he returned early from school, feeling really
rotten. As soon as he came in, he went to the bathroom and
was sick in the basin. His mother, alarmed, went through to
help and noticed a peculiar, sweetish, fruity smell – rather
like nail varnish remover. 'Glue!' she thought. 'He's been
sniffing glue.' Michael was breathing very rapidly and
deeply, and when he looked at her as if he didn't recognise
her, his mother became seriously alarmed and ran for
Michael's father.

One look was enough for Dad. 'I'm taking you to hospital'
he said, grimly.

Michael passed out completely on the way and was carried into the Casualty Department unconscious. The Casualty
officer sniffed his breath.

'Glue?' asked Michael's mother, anxiously.

The doctor didn't answer. 'Has he been drinking a lot?' he
asked.

'Yes. Far more than usual.'

'And passing a lot of urine?'

'Well, he's always in the toilet. I've heard him get up in the
night, too.'

The doctor was pushing a needle into a vein in Michael's
arm. 'Do you think he's been losing weight?' he asked.

'Yes, I think so.'

'What is it?' asked Michael's father. 'Why are you putting
up a drip?'

'Just a sec,' said the Casualty officer, adjusting the drip rate, in the chamber below the plastic bottle of saline. He took a narrow strip of paper from a jar and touched the end of it to a drop of blood near the needle in Michael's arm, looking at his watch as he did so.

Michael's father started to speak again, but the doctor silenced him with a glance and continued to look at his watch. After a minute, he picked up a wash bottle and carefully washed the blood off the end of the paper strip. Then he blotted it with a tissue and slipped it into a machine on the nearby bench. He stood looking at the read-out for a moment, then turned to Michael's parents.

'It's diabetic coma,' he said, quietly. 'He's desperately in need of insulin . . . and fluid.' He turned the control on the drip set so that the saline ran more quickly, and began to inject soluble insulin into the plastic tube.

That is an accurate account of an event that happens, with minor variations, somewhere in this country every day. About one young person in every thousand develops this kind of severe diabetes, requiring insulin for treatment. They don't all go into coma, of course, for in most cases it is clear, before that stage, that something is seriously wrong. You can learn a great deal about diabetes from this story – every point has significance (even the white stain on the trousers of Michael's pyjamas) – but before explaining, let me tell you another story.

Jennifer was forty-seven and had always had a problem with her weight. Her general health was pretty good, on the whole, but for several months she had been feeling exceptionally tired and had been annoyed, and dreadfully embarrassed, by a constant itching down below. The doctor called it 'pruritis' and said he suspected thrush. He had given her some pessaries, but they didn't seem to help. Her periods were irregular, too, and she was beginning to feel that she should ask for a referral to a gynaecologist, when something new came along to worry her.

She had been watching television and trying not to

11

scratch when, to her amazement, the picture and everything else at that end of the room became so blurred that she
could not make out any detail at all. Trying not to panic, she
picked up the *TV Times* and was surprised, and rather
relieved, to find that she could make out the print perfectly
clearly, without her reading glasses. She could even make it
out with the magazine held only a few inches from her eyes
– a thing she had not been able to do since she was an adolescent. To calm herself, she took a long swallow from her
pint glass of Coca-Cola.

Over the next day or two, Jennifer's vision seemed to
vary a little, but distance vision remained very blurred and it
was not long before she paid a visit to an optician for an eye
test. She thought the optician was very young, but he
seemed confident. After shining some lights at her eyes, he
put on a trial frame and slotted two lenses into place. 'How's
that?' he asked, indicating the test chart at the far end of the
room.

'Very good!' said Jennifer. 'I can read the bottom line.'

'You're short sighted,' said the optician. 'You have
myopia.'

'But it came on so suddenly. Is that usual?'

The young optician hesitated, then said uneasily, 'These
things happen.'

Jennifer chose a nice pair of frames and was told that her
glasses would be ready in ten days' time. But within a week
her vision had returned to normal and she needed her reading glasses again for close work.

When she went back to the optician and told him that she
could now see clearly in the distance, he looked embarrassed and an older man came across and said, 'Shall I see
this lady, Peter?' The young man turned pink and went
through to the office.

Jennifer's tests were repeated and they confirmed that
her distance vision was normal. She felt a bit sorry for the
young optician and said, 'I *was* short sighted. When I came
before, I couldn't read the chart – not without the lenses.
But now it's quite clear.'

The older man looked closely at her. 'Have you been

12

unusually thirsty recently?' he asked. 'I mean really thirsty?'

'Oh yes! For weeks!' said Jennifer, astonished. 'How on earth did you know?'

'I'm going to give you a note for your GP and I think you should see him as soon as possible. He'll explain it all to you.' He took a green form from a drawer and began to write on it.

'What about the glasses?' asked Jennifer.

'Forget it,' he said. 'You're not going to need them.'

When Jennifer's doctor read the optician's note, the probable connection between her tiredness, itchiness, thrush, visual disturbance and thirst at once became apparent and he sent her through to his nurse so that a sample of urine could be tested.

'Over two per cent of sugar,' reported the nurse.

You may be wondering how the same disease could affect two people so differently. Michael was losing weight rapidly, while Jennifer remained her usual tubby self. Michael went into a dangerous coma after only two or three weeks of illness, while Jennifer was able to carry on reasonably well for months. I will explain this shortly, but it will be more revealing if we consider, first, what it was that these two people had in common.

The most obvious thing was that when samples of their urine were tested they contained considerable quantities of glucose. Now this is quite abnormal. Glucose in the urine, except in very rare cases, must always be regarded seriously. This finding means that there is too much glucose in the blood and that is what we are really worried about. You are going to be hearing a lot about glucose, so we must take a look at this substance and at its importance to Michael and Jennifer – and to all of us.

About glucose

Glucose is a form of sugar – rather simpler than, and not quite so sweet as, ordinary cane sugar – and it is the essential fuel for the body, required for the normal functioning of

13

brain, muscles, nerves, glands – indeed of all our tissues. Glucose is just as much a fuel for the body as petrol is for a car. We store it and we 'burn' it – perhaps not quite so explosively as petrol is burned in a car, but the process is the same – a slow burning of fuel in oxygen. It is the burning of glucose that provides us with energy and keeps our bodies warm.

When I talk about 'sugar' in the body, I mean glucose. Without glucose we would quickly die, because our brains require an uninterrupted supply so that vital functions can continue. Fortunately, there is plenty of glucose in the body. Quite a high proportion of the food we eat gets broken down to glucose and we keep good stores in our livers and can convert stored protein and fat into glucose when the need arises.

But what about Michael's loss of weight? Isn't diabetes a wasting disease? And if there was so much fuel about, why should both Michael and Jennifer feel so weak and tired? Yes, diabetes is a wasting disease. Even the ancient Greek doctors knew this. Listen to what Arateus of Cappadocia said, nearly two thousand years ago: 'Diabetes isn't very common, but it's remarkable. The flesh just melts down into urine. The thirst is terrible and can't be quenched. Life is horrible . . . and short.' This description remained perfectly accurate until 1922, but, thanks to medical science, it no longer applies. At the turn of the century, Michael would have had no chance at all. He would certainly have died. Jennifer might possibly have survived, if she could have stuck to a rigid diet. But, let's be realistic, the most likely outcome is that she would have eaten herself to death.

The explanation is that, in diabetes, the fuel, glucose, can't get into the tissue cells to be used. The glucose which is absorbed quite normally through the intestines, after a meal, simply accumulates in the blood. Not only that, but the fuel stores, in the muscles and in the fat deposits under the skin, are not able to retain their fuel. It just leaks out, the liver is forced to convert the stored material into glucose, and the amount of glucose dissolved in the blood gets greater and greater until the blood contains many times the

14

normal amount. This considerable rise in the amount of sugar in the blood never happens to a non-diabetic person. In a healthy person an unnecessary rise in the blood sugar immediately leads to the storage of glucose – in the liver and muscles and in the fat deposits.

But Michael and Jennifer, for reasons that will soon be clear to you, were unable to store their glucose properly, and the quantity in their blood rose to abnormally high levels. I expect you know that the kidneys act to keep the amounts of most of the substances in the blood within reasonable limits. In health, glucose is too valuable to waste, so, at normal blood sugar levels, none of it passes through the kidneys into the urine. Healthy people almost never have sugar in their urine. But when the amount of glucose in the blood rises above a certain point the kidneys start leaking it through and the urine becomes sweet. Physicians used to diagnose diabetes by tasting the urine, and they gave the name *diabetes mellitus* to the condition. 'Mellitus' comes from the Latin word 'mel' meaning honey.

Michael had so much sugar in his urine that when a splash dried out on his pyjamas, the sugar crystals were left behind. And some of that sugar came from Michael's muscles and from the fat that had previously rounded out his figure.

So what is it about Michael and Jennifer that stops them from storing away their excess sugar in an orderly manner? And why did Michael's breath smell like nail varnish remover? I'm going to answer these questions in the next two chapters, but rather than leave you with too many riddles, let me explain some of the other symptoms experienced by our two diabetics.

Why are untreated diabetics so thirsty?

Our kidneys are marvellous organs with a remarkable ability to regulate the amounts of various substances in the blood. But when faced with the kind of levels of sugar encountered in untreated diabetes, they have problems. Obviously, they are going to try to get rid of as much of the surplus sugar as possible, but if they were to do this using the normal rate of urine production, the urine would be like syrup and the sugar might even crystallize out in the kidneys or the bladder. So to get rid of a lot of sugar, the kidneys need a lot of water and they can get this only from the blood. So in diabetes the kidneys must produce much more than the normal amount of urine (causing poor Michael to have to get up two or three times each night) and, in the process, the blood loses a great deal of water and gets concentrated. It is this shortage of water that causes the thirst.

Naturally, the thirst leads to an unusually high intake of water, in the form of squashes, coffee, tea, Coke, etc., but this extra water is immediately excreted by the kidneys, in their attempt to dilute the sugar which is being passed.

What about the itch?

Jennifer's GP was quite right about her itching being due to thrush, although he was a bit slow off the mark in appreciating why she had it. Thrush is a fungus infection caused by a mould called *candida albicans*. This spreading nasty thrives in warm, moist, dark places and one thing that will encourage its enthusiastic growth is plenty of sugar. As we have seen, Jennifer was more than moderately obliging in this respect. As a matter of fact, male diabetics, too, often get an itch down below, for very similar reasons. This is more likely in uncircumcised men, who often develop an inflammation of the bulb of the penis (the 'glans') as a result of candida infection. This is called *balanitis* and it may cause severe discomfort.

Other symptoms

Jennifer's tiredness is easy to explain. Although she had plenty of fuel, she wasn't able to use any of it properly, so the full amount of energy, which should have been provided by the burning of the glucose, simply wasn't available to her.

But what about the strange story of the temporary short

sight? You now know that uncontrolled diabetes results in a high level of sugar in the blood. All the tissues of the body have to be intimately surrounded by blood or by fluid derived from the blood, because it is the blood that supplies them with fuel, and the oxygen with which to burn it. Among these tissues are the focussing lenses inside our eyes; and the shape and curvature of these lenses are readily modified by alteration in the amount of substances dissolved in the fluid that surrounds them. Changes in the blood sugar levels lead to such alterations and this, in turn, alters the power of the lenses. This is why the vision tends to be affected by untreated diabetes. The commonest lens change is an increase in curvature, so that the light is bent more strongly and the rays come to a focus in front of the retina. In this condition, the only rays which can focus on the retina are those coming from near objects – hence the short sight.

So now you understand quite a lot about what diabetes is and how it affects people. But to have any real working knowledge of diabetes, you are going to have to learn a good deal more than that. And basic to your understanding will be an appreciation of the central role of the substance called 'insulin'. Insulin is so important that I have given it an entire chapter to itself. First, however, let's look at the reasons why some people become diabetics.

2 WHAT CAUSES IT?

High up inside your abdomen, and lying along the back wall, immediately behind your stomach, is your pancreas. This is a gland, about 6in long, and from it a duct runs into your duodenum. The most obvious function of your pancreas is to manufacture a powerful digestive juice which actively breaks down the meat you eat into simpler, and more easily absorbed substances. Every time you eat protein, your pancreas squirts some of this juice into your bowel, the acid from your stomach is neutralised and the protein begins to be digested so that its products can be assimilated and used as 'building bricks' for body maintenance and growth.

But the pancreas has a second, and quite independent function. Scattered throughout the substance of the gland are little islands of cells, quite different from those which produce the digestive juice. These islets of cells are so important that they are given the name 'The Islets of Langerhans' after the man, Paul Langerhans, who discovered them. The islet cells also produce a powerful substance, but this time, instead of releasing the product into the bowel, they release it into the blood stream. The stuff they manufacture is one of a group of substances called 'Hormones' and this hormone, because it comes from islands and because the Latin word for an island is 'Insula', is called 'Insulin'.

Diabetes is all about insulin. Diabetics are people who can't produce their own insulin, or can't produce enough of it to meet the needs of their bodies, and if you understand insulin and its actions, you will understand diabetes. So you must expect to find quite a lot about insulin in this book – how its production is controlled, how it operates in the body, the effects of too little and too much, the relationship of insulin to food intake, and so on. By the time you have read this book, you will be quite an expert on insulin – and, as a diabetic, that is certainly what you ought to be.

I expect you have decided by now that diabetics have something wrong with their pancreases. In the case of severe 'insulin-dependent' diabetics (people who depend on insulin injections for the maintenance of their health) that is quite true, but, as we shall see, not all diabetics have malfunctioning pancreases. Indeed there are some diabetics who produce quite normal amounts of insulin. But don't let this confuse you. All will be explained shortly. The study of diabetes has much to do with the relationship of one thing to another – such as the differing amounts of insulin needed by people of differing weight, or the effects on insulin requirement of varying food intake or amount of exercise. These are things you are going to have to understand, but, happily, none of them is really difficult. If you just keep at it steadily, it will all become clear.

You are quite right in thinking that the pancreases of people with severe diabetes don't produce insulin and, as you infer, it is the problem with their pancreases that causes the diabetes. So let's take a look, first, at what it is that goes wrong with the pancreas. Once we get this out of the way, we can get down to a study of insulin.

The cause of diabetes

I expect you are wondering why, in some people, the Islet cells of the pancreas should stop producing insulin. Well, I'm wondering too. The truth is that no one knows, for certain, why this should happen. There are plenty of guesses, some of them based on very suggestive evidence. There is, for instance, definite proof that when diabetes occurs in schoolchildren, the onset is three times as common in the wintertime than in the summer. The same kind of frequency applies to certain virus infections and a few cases have

19

actually been proved in which the Islets of Langerhans have been damaged by such viruses.

But there is also definite evidence that, although this kind of diabetes is not wholly caused by a genetic factor, there is certainly an inherited susceptibility to it. A third factor known to be important is the way in which the individual's natural body defences react to virus infections. At the present stage of medical knowledge, it seems likely that the damage to the Islet cells occurs as a result of a virus infection which is dangerous only to those with the hereditary tendency. This is no more than an inspired guess and it may be overthrown at any moment by advances in medical research.

Such research is, of course, vitally important. Suppose, for instance, that it could be established that the Islet damage is in fact caused, as some scientists believe, by Coxackie B4 virus infection of susceptible people. The next stage would, of course, be to prepare a vaccine against this virus and to give it to susceptible individuals so that they might be immunised against diabetes. I certainly don't want to seem to be suggesting that a vaccine against diabetes is just around the corner. This is unlikely, for the subject of diabetes, at a research level, is immensely complicated and although a great deal has been discovered, the whole solution is not yet within our grasp.

Twin studies

There is strong evidence that late-onset diabetes is a hereditary disease and we know that, in many of these cases, there is no damage to the Islets of Langerhans. As we shall see in a moment, obesity plays an important part in the development of this type of diabetes. There are some cases, however, in which it can be proved that the genetic factor acts by causing interference with the production of insulin.

Studies of identical twins with diabetes are of enormous interest, because such twins have identical chromosomes. These studies have shown that, in the group of twins over forty years of age, if one twin develops diabetes, the other will almost always also contract the disease. But when we look at young twins, one of whom has become diabetic, we find that the other has a much smaller chance of developing the disease. This finding confirms that the causes of many cases of maturity-onset diabetes are different from those of juvenile, insulin-dependent diabetes.

Obesity

Careful statistical studies have proved that, in the older age groups, diabetes is much commoner in fat people than in thin. Indeed, at least half of all the people diagnosed as having maturity-onset diabetes are obese. Does this mean that the obesity causes the diabetes? Let's consider what happened to Jennifer after the astute optician realised that she was a diabetic.

Her GP referred her to an excellent diabetic clinic where, in addition to having the type of her diabetes sorted out and appropriate treatment prescribed, she agreed to take part in a scientific study which was going on into the causes of late-onset diabetes. The doctor, who was a member of the team doing this work, was especially keen to have her in the trial because she was, by any standards, considerably overweight.

So, in addition to having frequent urine tests for sugar, and many measurements of the amount of sugar in her blood, Jennifer was also investigated for the levels of insulin in her blood at various times of the day and following differing amounts of food intake. Insulin levels are not so easy to measure as sugar levels and this is not a test which is done routinely. If such a test were done in a severe diabetic, it would, of course, show either a complete absence of insulin or only very low levels. Surprisingly, Jennifer's blood insulin levels were, on every occasion, notably *higher* than the insulin levels of a normal healthy person of normal weight!

While at the clinic, Jennifer became friendly with a Margery, a married woman of about her own age, also very much on the rotund pattern. 'How long have you been diabetic?' asked Jennifer.

'I'm not.'

'Not diabetic? Then what are you doing here?'

21

'My daughter's an audio-typist in the hospital. They wanted volunteers, on the . . . stout side, for this trial, and she told me about it. So I said I would do it.'

'What are they doing to you?'

'Blood sugar, blood insulin – you know.'

In fact, considerable numbers of volunteers were being checked and Jennifer and Margery were typical of what they were finding. Fat people, whether maturity-onset diabetics or not, nearly always had high insulin levels. This was not surprising, in the non-diabetics, because as we know, the amount of insulin produced by the pancreas is carefully regulated in accordance with the amounts of sugar in the blood and, of course, fat people always have more sugar in the blood than normal. But what was especially interesting was that one could be a diabetic while still having plenty of insulin in the blood.

How to cure diabetes

This trial showed that although many maturity-onset diabetics had more insulin in the blood than normal people of normal weight, they had rather less than non-diabetic people who were as fat as they were. Jennifer and Margery were equally fat and both had higher than normal levels of insulin in their blood, but Jennifer, who was diabetic, had less insulin than Margery – who was not.

In fact, a good deal of progress has been made since that trial was done, and we now know that when insulin attaches itself to the surface of body cells it can do so only at certain places called 'insulin receptors'. Studies have shown that obese, maturity-onset diabetics have fewer of these receptors than normal people, so although they may have plenty of insulin in the blood, only some of it can find places to attach itself. This state is known as 'insulin resistance'. And what is quite fascinating about this, and of the greatest importance to all obese maturity-onset diabetics, is that if such people can get their weight down, by establishing new eating habits, the number of insulin receptors increases, the blood insulin levels drop along with the glucose levels, and the diabetes may be cured!

3 ALL ABOUT INSULIN

Insulin is a very complex chemical. A man called Frederick Sanger worked for eight years in a Cambridge laboratory to sort out the chemical structure. He finally succeeded in 1953 and they gave him the Nobel Prize. This was richly deserved and the work had important consequences for diabetics, leading to methods of converting ox or pig insulin (to which some diabetic people are allergic) into human insulin. You will learn more about this later. Insulin is complex because it has a complex biochemical function in the body, but it isn't necessary to understand biochemistry to understand how it works, and, as you will see in a moment, the matter is really quite simple to grasp.

Insulin manufactured in the Islet cells goes directly into the blood-stream and is at once carried by the circulation to all parts of the body. In the normal person, the amount of insulin produced is automatically regulated by the amount of glucose in the blood. The higher the glucose levels, the more insulin produced. This control occurs in the pancreas itself, which responds to raised glucose levels, in the blood passing through it, by producing more insulin.

Insulin attaches itself to the outer surface of nearly all the cells of the body – muscle cells, fat cells, skin, heart, abdominal organs – and forms a sort of one-way channel system which allows the glucose in the blood to get in. If there is a lot of glucose in the blood, the resulting increased quantity of insulin opens up a lot of new ports to allow the surplus glucose to get into the tissue cells to be stored or used as fuel. But what if there isn't any insulin, or not enough? Well, in that case there are no inlet channels and, while plenty of glucose is accumulating in the blood, the muscles and other tissues are starved of fuel and have no alternative but to feed upon their own substance. That is why, although there is plenty of fuel (glucose) in the blood – indeed often much too much – the muscles just waste away in diabetes.

The matter is a little more complicated than this, because there are hormones, such as adrenaline and cortico-steroids, and a substance called 'glucagon' which are all constantly acting to break down fuel stores and release glucose into the blood. Normally, loss of glucose from the tissues, as a result of this, is quickly made up by the return of glucose from the blood into the cells. But if, as a result of a shortage or absence of insulin, glucose can't get into the cells, wasting of the tissues will, of course, be rapid. That, in essence, is how insulin works. And now you can see how the essential features of diabetes come about – the excess sugar in the blood, spilling over into the urine; the progressive and rapid loss of weight; the wasting of the muscles; the weakness. And now you can, I hope, better understand the things that were happening to the people in the little stories I have been telling.

Our three characters, Michael, Jennifer and Margery all have an insulin problem. Michael doesn't manufacture any, and so he is an 'insulin-dependent' diabetic – that is, he is dependent on injections of insulin to keep him alive and healthy. Jennifer's pancreas does produce insulin – quite a lot, in fact – more than most people, although not quite so much as Margery – but not quite enough to keep down the levels of sugar in her blood. Moreover, the insulin she does produce isn't all able to be used because of the reduced number of insulin receptor sites on the surfaces of her tissue cells. Margery produces a great deal of insulin – indeed, quite a worrying amount, and one wonders if the Islets of Langerhans in her pancreas are going to be able to keep up this high demand. But, so far, she has been able to produce enough insulin to cope with the large quantities of sugar released into her blood.

Insulin is, of course, a chemical substance and obviously has powerful properties. It is a protein, and meat (muscle) is made of protein. But, in muscle, the protein molecules ('building bricks') all stick together to form a large, visible mass. The molecules of insulin, manufactured as separate units in the 'Beta' cells of the Islets of Langerhans, slip straight into the blood, like a huge shoal of invisible eels and are carried all around the body to search for, and attach themselves to, their receptor sites on the cell membranes of muscle, fat, nerve and other tissues.

Why can't we take insulin by mouth?

The fact that insulin is a protein has a very important practical consequence, especially for people like Michael. Because he can't produce any himself, Michael must get his insulin from outside. That's clear enough. But why inject it? Why doesn't he just swallow a little from time to time? This would be a lot less trouble and grief than having to stick needles into himself twice a day.

Protein in our diet can't be absorbed immediately into the blood-stream, because the molecules are too big. So all of it has to go through a digestive process to break it down into molecules of more manageable size (amino acids). Unfortunately, insulin taken by mouth would be treated, in the bowel, in exactly the same way as rump steak, and long before it was absorbed into the blood-stream, it wouldn't be insulin any more. Ironically, the stuff that turns protein into simpler and readily absorbable substances comes from the pancreas! Whenever protein is eaten the pancreas carries out its other function and squirts some protein-digesting juice into the duodenum. So it's no good trying to take insulin by mouth.

The controlling effect of insulin

First, let me tell you what happens in the normal person with normal insulin production. We have seen that the amount of insulin produced at any time is accurately matched to the level of sugar in the blood. And we have also seen that insulin attaches itself to the outer membranes of muscle, fat, skin and other cells of the body so as to allow glucose to pass from the blood into them. Equally important, it also stops glucose from leaking out again. When we eat a meal, sugar floods into the blood-stream from the digested carbohydrate (sugars, starches, bread, potatoes etc.) and this supply of glucose continues for about two hours. Some of this sugar is immediately used up for normal energy needs.

The rise in the blood sugar level, of course, prompts the pancreas to manufacture more insulin. This, in turn, causes the surplus sugar to be stored in the muscles and, in an altered form, in fat cells. Surplus sugar is also stored in the liver in the form of a 'polymer' of glucose – that is, lots of glucose molecules linked together, in much the same way that ethylene molecules are linked together to form poly-thene. This 'polyglucose' is called 'glycogen' and the liver glycogen store provides a readily available source of glucose for use when energy is needed between meals. Interest-ingly, in a real emergency, when we need lots of fuel quickly, the adrenaline which is always produced on these occasions, actually forces the liver to break off the mol-ecules of glucose from the glycogen and these are freed into the blood-stream.

But the liver can't store a great deal of glycogen – about 120 grams – and this will provide only about 500 calories, which is not very much. Someone leading a normal quiet life might use up 2000 calories a day. So, unless we eat carbohy-drates at regular intervals, the glycogen is soon used up and glucose has to be got from somewhere else.

How the body makes its own sugar

Now the liver is a remarkable organ with an impressive capacity for chemical engineering. It can do surprising things with glucose, apart from forming glycogen, and has the ability to turn it into fat. It does this when we have eaten more than we need for our immediate energy require-ments, and that is why we get fat when we eat too much – even the carbohydrates get turned into fat, and are laid down in the fat stores under the skin and in the abdomen.

But the liver also has the surprising ability to manufacture sugar, and when we don't eat any carbohydrate or when we starve ourselves, this is what it does. The process is called '*gluconeogenesis*' ('neo' means 'new' and 'genesis' means 'birth') and it is important that you should know about it. The new glucose is made, in the liver, from the constituents of protein. These are called 'amino acids'. Suppose we were to live on an exclusive diet of fillet steak. We would still need a lot of glucose, because glucose is the basic body fuel, and the liver, 'aware' that sugar levels were low, would turn to the amino acids which were being absorbed from the gut after the steak had been digested by the pancreatic juice. For the liver to carry out the process of turning amino acids into sugar, energy is required, and as the normal fuel for this – glucose – isn't available, the liver uses fat which it gets from the dietary input (unless you have cut the fat off the steak) or from the body's fat stores.

Ketone bodies

But fat doesn't burn up cleanly, as glucose does, to produce only water and carbon dioxide. Burning fat produces substances called 'ketone bodies', one of which is acetone. You can, if you like, think of ketone bodies as a kind of 'smoky exhaust' produced by the burning of fat. But, in fact, these ketone bodies are quite useful, in the healthy person, as they can, up to a point, be used outside the liver as a general fuel. The brain, for instance, is quite happy to run on ketone bodies, in moderate quantities. Normally, the amount of sugar produced by gluconeogenesis, and the quantity of ketone bodies released into the blood, are limited by the built-in controlling effect of insulin. As soon as the blood sugar levels rise, more insulin is produced and this slows down the rate of gluconeogenesis.

What happens in starvation? Well, of course, nothing is arriving from the gut and both the ingredients and the fuel for the manufacture of glucose (the amino acids and the fats) have to be obtained from the body's own stores. Because the blood sugar levels are low, in starvation, there will, of course, be very little insulin circulating, and we have seen that low insulin levels allow easy release of protein (amino acids) from the muscles and fat from the fat stores. So the muscles waste and the fat stores get used up in the interests of maintaining the essential supply of glucose, without which we would quickly die. Ketone bodies are, of course, produced in starvation.

Now let's consider what happens in diabetes. Without insulin, there is a constant flow of protein (amino acids) from the muscles, and fat from the fat deposits – just as happens in starvation, but in a much bigger way – and, of course, the liver gets flooded with these substances. The result, naturally, is that it immediately gets down to a great effort of gluconeogenesis and there is a tremendous outpouring of new glucose into the blood. But at the same time, because of the burning of so much fat in the liver, there is an equally excessive flow of ketone bodies into the blood. The acetone, one of the ketones, being volatile, passes out in the lungs and appears in the breath. It was this that made Michael's breath smell like nail varnish remover, and caused his mother to suspect that he had been glue-sniffing. But this is not very important. What really matters is that ketone bodies are acidic in nature and, if present in sufficient quantities, will turn the blood acid. This is extremely dangerous, can easily cause coma, and may be fatal.

A recap on insulin action

The action of insulin is admittedly rather complicated, but it is so important for you to understand it that I am going to repeat the main points for you in the form of a summary.

- A rise in blood sugar causes a rise in insulin production by the pancreas. A fall in blood sugar causes less insulin to be produced.
- Insulin attaches itself to the surface of the body cells and forms 'valves' which allow glucose to enter, but not to leave, the cells.

- If there is a shortage of insulin, the glucose can't get into the cells, but whatever is inside can easily get out. This applies especially to muscle cells and fat storage cells.
- In the case of muscle cells, the absence of insulin allows the amino acids – the constituents of muscle protein – to leak out easily into the blood.
- Likewise, in the case of fat cells, shortage of insulin leads to a considerable quantity of fat passing out of the cells into the blood.
- Insulin encourages the liver to store glucose as 'glycogen' – which is a convenient form of glucose storage for use between meals.
- If there is a shortage of blood glucose, the resulting low insulin levels prompt the liver to start to produce new glucose, using amino acids as constituents and fat as fuel. This is called 'gluconeogenesis'.
- A by-product of 'gluconeogenesis' is a group of substances called 'ketone bodies'. These are fine in moderation, but can be disastrous in excess.
- In diabetes, the absence of insulin causes uncontrolled gluconeogenesis to occur, even in the presence of large quantities of sugar.
- The process liberates ketone bodies and these release acetone in the lungs which gives the breath a characteristic smell. Severe ketosis may alter the acidity of the blood and can kill.

Michael's case analysed

We can now understand, more clearly, what happened to Michael. We still don't know what it was that damaged the 'Beta' cells in the Islets of Langerhans in his pancreas, but we do know that over the course of only a few weeks, his pancreas stopped producing insulin. As a result, his muscles were unable to use the glucose from his blood and their protein started to break down and leak amino acids. At the same time, Michael was unable to store glucose in the form of fat and his fat stores were also soon depleted. So his muscles began to waste away, he felt weak and lacking in energy, and his clothes became very loose. The amino acids and fats were carried around in the blood and passed into his liver where they were immediately converted (by gluconeogenesis) into the very thing he didn't need – more glucose.

Partly because of his inability to use up glucose and partly because of the gluconeogenesis, the level of sugar in Michael's blood rose higher and higher. This, in itself, didn't do very much harm (although excess sugar in the tissues can cause a variety of problems, including a tendency to infection) but as the level of sugar rose it soon reached the point at which Michael's kidneys were forced to try to get rid of the surplus. So lots of sugar began to appear in his urine and, to keep the concentration down, his kidneys had to extract extra water from his blood. This meant large volumes of urine output and great thirst.

Eventually the 'ketone body' production (secondary to gluconeogenesis) reached a level at which Michael's mother could smell the acetone on his breath, and soon the resulting severe disturbance of all his normal body biochemical processes led to brain malfunction and coma.

Where does medicinal insulin come from?

You will now appreciate that insulin is an important substance, and you will want to know how medicinal insulin is obtained. For many years now, it has been obtained from the pancreases of oxen and pigs. These two insulins are not exactly identical to human insulin or to each other, and pig's insulin is closer, in chemical structure, to human, than is ox insulin. So, for as long as these were the only source of supply, pig's insulin was to be preferred. The reasons for this will become apparent when we discuss insulin antibodies.

Although pig insulin is pretty close in structure to human insulin, some people react badly even to it and a great deal of research has been done to try to convert it to the exact structure of human insulin. This was achieved at the end of the 1970s and insulin, converted from porcine insulin, and having the exact chemical composition of human insulin, is now available. But the scientists have gone further. Insulin has now actually been synthesised – that is, the complex protein molecule has been put together from simpler groups of atoms. By 1977 enough synthetic human insulin had been made to enable the workers to carry out a series of clinical trials with it. But making insulin this way is difficult and expensive and, at about the same time, a new and very exciting development occurred which rather put synthesis in the shade.

Insulin by genetic engineering

This is an almost incredible process. I expect you know that every cell in our body contains a kind of 'programme' for all our physical characteristics. This programme is in the form of very complex molecules called 'chromosomes', made of stuff called DNA, and each chromosome carries many local sub-programmes called genes. The genes are, in fact, the programmes for the production of protein and each gene can cause the cell to manufacture a particular protein. There is, therefore, a gene for insulin, and whenever this gene is present, and is 'switched on', insulin will be produced.

Now genes can do this in cells other than human cells and, a few years ago, scientists managed to introduce human genes for insulin into the single-cell bodies of bacteria called *E. coli*. As soon as they did this the bugs started to manufacture tiny quantities of human insulin. That was remarkable enough, but there was more to come. Having successfully solved this extraordinarily complex problem, the scientists, as they anticipated, had an incredible bonus. The bacteria which had accepted the new gene and survived, now had a different chromosome from before and, in the natural course of events, this altered chromosome would be inherited by every single future descendant of these bacteria. And, of course, all these 'clones', as they are called, would be identical to the altered progenitor, and all of them would manufacture insulin.

So, once the insulin gene had been successfully implanted, all that was necessary was to give the bugs the kind of living conditions they like best, and plenty of food, and they reproduced like mad. You can culture tons of them, if you like. The problems haven't all been solved yet, but the method seems almost certain to be the future answer to the production of pure human insulin (see Ch. 13, p. 000).

4 TREATMENT BY DIET AND TABLETS

At the diabetic clinic, Jennifer weighed in at 204 lbs – a real heavyweight. At 5 ft 6 in, her ideal weight was around 124 lbs, so there was a surplus of 80 lbs, which must have cost her a lot of insulin to lay down and maintain. The doctor didn't make any cracks about her weight, but she knew what he was thinking and she asked him outright whether her weight was the cause of her diabetes.

'Very likely,' said the doctor.

'But I hardly eat anything!' said Jennifer.

The doctor's face relaxed a little. 'Drink tea, do you?'

'Oh yes. I'm fond of a cuppa.'

'How many cups a day?'

Jennifer considered. 'Oh, I don't know. Quite a few.'

'Ten?'

Jennifer thought of the two or three cups before breakfast and the three or four with the meal, then the mid-morning cup or three. . . 'More like twenty,' she said.

'How many spoons of sugar?'

'Three,' said Jennifer, guiltily.

The doctor nodded and seemed to change the subject. 'You remember we asked you to eat nothing for twelve hours before we took the first blood sample and gave you the sugary drink?'

'Yes.'

'Did you drink any tea that morning? Before coming here?'

'No.'

'Good. Right. That test was what we call a glucose tolerance test. The blood samples we took every half hour

33

were analysed to see what your blood sugar was doing.'

'And what did it show?'

'Well, the normal range is from about 3 to 7. The high figure comes about an hour after eating and should drop again to 3 or 4, after another hour.' (See p. 00 for fuller explanation of numbers.)

'What did I have?' asked Jennifer.

'You hit the ceiling,' said the doctor, seriously. 'After two hours, the level was still nearly 20.'

'Is that bad?'

'Of course it's bad! But I'm not surprised, the way you've been going on. Now listen. You're diabetic. But you're still producing plenty of insulin. Quite enough for any normal person of your height. You're giving yourself diabetes. Do you realise that without eating a single solid mouthful – and I guarantee you eat quite a few – you're taking in 300 grams of pure sugar a day in your tea. That's 1200 calories – enough to live on – and it's probably only about a quarter of your total intake.'

Jennifer felt bad, and longed for a cup of tea. She didn't think the doctor was very sympathetic and wondered if he had ever had to try to lose weight.

'You're going to cut out sugar – completely,' said the doctor.

Jennifer paled.

'And no jam, no marmalade, no syrup, no treacle, no honey. Nothing sweet at all. Drink as much tea as you like, but NO SUGAR. You're to eat no chocolate, no chocolate biscuits, no sweet cakes or biscuits, no buns, no eclairs, no meringues, no pastry, no sweets of any kind, no syrupy tinned fruit, no sweet drinks——'

Jennifer started to get up. 'Are you trying to kill me?' she asked.

'Sit down,' said the doctor. 'I'm trying to cure you. There are plenty of other things you can eat – things you will come to enjoy, in time. There's a very good chance that if you are sensible and change your eating habits, we can cure your diabetes. And you'll feel – and look – a lot better.'

'But I must have carbohydrates——'protested Jennifer.

'Certainly. You need plenty of carbohydrate. But not that kind. Let me tell you about fibre.'

Reluctantly, Jennifer listened as the doctor explained that foods rich in fibre released their sugar slowly so that even diabetics could have a blood sugar curve, after eating, that was quite close to normal; that fibre in the diet could trap cholesterol and other fats and carry them through the bowel so that one had the pleasure of eating them without the resulting pain of storing them. He told her that insulin-dependent diabetics who took their carbohydrates in the form of high-fibre foods could nearly always manage on smaller doses of insulin.

Jennifer did not feel very enthusiastic about all this. 'If I were to cut out the sweet things,' she asked, 'couldn't I just get by on protein and fats?'

The doctor looked at her over the top of his glasses. 'You'd find it expensive,' he said, bluntly, 'and you'd probably end up with a coronary thrombosis. Thin, non-diabetic women have considerable immunity, but people like you . . .'

Jennifer started to cry, but the doctor seemed unmoved. 'I could be nice to you,' he said, 'and tell you the things you want to hear. It would be a lot easier on me, too, I assure you. But it would probably be disastrous for you. So mop up and listen. It's the health food shop for you. Wholemeal, stone-ground bread, potatoes in their jackets, brown rice, oat cakes, porridge oats, raw vegetables, fruit, beans . . .'

Jennifer got the message and, although she had a bad time for several weeks, she managed, in spite of everything, to follow the doctor's advice. After six months she look remarkably trim – quite attractive, in fact – and felt marvellous. The glucose tolerance test was repeated and the result, although not entirely normal, was nearly so – the level peaked at 11 and two hours after the glucose drink it was down to 6. Regular testing of her urine showed that it was permanently free from sugar. But, in spite of this, her blood insulin measurements showed that she was now producing markedly less than she had at the height of her illness, indicating that her body's need for insulin was now much reduced.

The different forms of diabetes

Jennifer's case is obviously very different from Michael's. Because Michael's pancreas is not producing any insulin at all, the only way he can be kept well is to have insulin. Diet alone – even a starvation diet – could not save him. But there is a third type of diabetes – also usually occurring later in life – in which the person concerned is producing insulin but in which even conscientious dieting will not, by itself, control the disease. Of course, there are plenty of fat diabetic people like Jennifer, who could be free of the disease if they could bring themselves to lose weight and stick to a sensible diet, but who, for various reasons, are unable to do so.

I think we have to acknowledge that, to many people, eating is one of the most important things in life. And however clearly we may see the harm these people are doing themselves, we must recognise the strength of this impulse and respect their right to live in this way. So the third group of diabetics will also contain many people of this sort. It is a very large group and constitutes the great majority of diabetics.

So our three types of diabetics are:

- Non-insulin producing, insulin-dependent diabetics
- Insulin-producing, diet-controlled diabetics
- Insulin-producing diabetics, who cannot (or will not) be controlled by diet

It is this third group to whom I now turn.

Treatment by tablets

'Will it be the needles or the pills, doctor?' is a perennial question every GP is familiar with. And, happily, the answer, in the great majority of cases, is 'the pills'. So what are these magic tablets and how do they work?

The story goes back to the days before penicillin and the other antibiotics were generally available. In those days, doctors treating infection had to rely on a class of drugs called sulphonamides, of which one of the most successful early examples was M. & B. 693. Older readers will remember the sensation May and Baker caused by the introduction of this, the first of the 'wonder drugs'. About 1930, it was noted that the sulphonamides could lower blood sugar, but no one paid much attention until, in 1942, a French doctor, Marcel Janbon, who was treating patients with sulphonamides, for typhoid fever, was horrified when three of them died, not from the disease but from hypoglycaemia. This is the condition in which the blood sugar is too low, and you will learn all about it in Chapter 7.

The observation that these drugs could lower the blood sugar led to research into this effect and to the development of a range of drugs in which this action was especially strong. The most effective of these drugs are called the 'sulphonylureas' and they form the mainstay of the treatment of diabetes in people who are still producing insulin.

How do the tablets work?

When sulphonylureas are given to people like Michael – people not producing any insulin – nothing happens. The blood sugar is unaffected and the patient doesn't get any better. But if a normal person is given a tablet of Chlorpropamide ('Diabenese') or Tolbutamide ('Rastinon') there is an immediate increase in the production of insulin and the blood sugar levels drop, just as would happen if we gave a normal person an injection of insulin. This could, of course, be dangerous, and no one in their right senses would give sulphonylureas to normal people. But in mild diabetics, who are not producing quite enough insulin, the effect can obviously be extremely valuable.

It seem clear that, in some way, the drugs are succeeding in stimulating the Islets of Langerhans to secrete more insulin than they normally can. As may perhaps be expected, they don't seem to be able to do this indefinitely, and after about six months the action on the Islets is usually lost. One might expect, from this, that the drugs would then be totally ineffective. But, surprisingly, the insulin-stimulating effect is not the only action of these remarkable drugs. Several other effects have been found. The sulphonylureas reduce the amount of glucose absorbed from the gut after a carbohydrate meal; they reduce the rate of release of glucose from the liver by making it harder for the liver to release glucose molecules from stored glycogen; they interfere with the liver's ability to manufacture new glucose ('gluconeogenesis') and they act on the Alpha cells of the Islets to reduce the production of Glucagon (see Ch. 3).

All this means that even when the drugs no longer prompt increased insulin production, they may still be highly effective in controlling mild diabetes.

Can they be dangerous?

In answering this question we must consider a factor which has nothing to do with the drugs themselves. I have mentioned that quite a lot of people, who ought to 'cure' their diabetes by getting their weight down and establishing new and healthier eating habits, are able to carry on eating themselves to death by virtue of these tablets. A very well-known large American study of the effect of these drugs, published in 1970, and known as the University Group Diabetes Program seemed to show that there was a higher mortality rate, especially from heart disease, among those taking diabetes tablets, than among those having insulin or dummy tablets. Like most statistics, the results were open to various interpretations and the arguments still haven't been settled. But the American doctors took them seriously enough to cut down considerably on prescribing these drugs. British and European doctors were not sufficiently impressed to alter their practice very much.

There is, however, one clear lesson from all this – it is very much better to control one's diabetes, if one can, by weight loss and diet, than by any form of drug treatment. The figures for mortality among the people taking the dummy tablets were surprisingly low. Obviously, the American doctors, in setting up the trials, must have selected for that group those patients whom they thought could manage safely without drugs.

The sulphonylureas do have some side effects and the most important, and common, of these is an undue drop in the blood sugar level (hypoglycaemia). This may happen if the drugs are taken in excessive dosage or without due regard to the amount of food eaten. But I shall be dealing with the important matter of hypoglycaemia in Chapter 7.

Another side effect is a skin rash, all over the body, starting soon after one of these drugs is first given. This is an allergy and may occasionally be dangerous, so the doctor will probably stop the drug. Skin rashes are not very common – perhaps one in every fifty patients taking sulphonylurea drugs will suffer it. Rarely, very severe skin eruptions may occur.

An odd, and quite common, reaction to this group of drugs is flushing of the face after drinking a little alcohol. This may be embarrassing to the person concerned and has been known to put people off alcohol altogether. This is not usually necessary, but in some people taking one of this group of drugs – Diabinese – alcohol causes severe nausea and even vomiting.

Other diabetes tablets

The sulphonylurea group, although the most important, are not the only tablets used in the control of diabetes. The other main group contains the drugs called the 'biguanides'. These have no pancreas-stimulating effect and work in a manner similar to the secondary actions of the sulphonylureas. But they have some major disadvantages and must be used with care.

Diabetics on treatment by tablets are often confused by the names of these drugs and, as there are at least three names for each, this is not surprising. For those who like to know what they are taking, there follows a table giving the 'approved' names, and a few of the trade names, of the commoner drugs.

39

Sulphonylurea drugs

'Approved' name	Trade name
Acetohexamide	(Dimelor)
Chlorpropamide	(Diabinese, Glymese, Melitase)
Glibenclamide	(Daonil, Semi-daonil, Euglucon)
Glibornuride	(Glutril)
Gliclazide	(Diamicron)
Glipizide	(Glibenese, Minodiab)
Gliquidone	Glurenorm
Glymidine	(Gondafon)
Tolazamide	(Tolanase)
Tolbutamide	(Pramidex, Rastinon)

Biguanide drugs

'Approved name'	Trade name
Metformin	(Glucophage, Metiguanide)
Phenformin	(Dibotin, Dipar)

5 DIET AND BLOOD SUGAR

This chapter is mainly for insulin-dependent diabetics, but please don't skip it just because you are on tablets, for it also contains much that concerns you. It is important to understand that although your doctor, or the people at the diabetic clinic, can advise and help you, the responsibility, in the end, has to remain with you. However well he may have advised you, your doctor doesn't really know how much, or what, you are eating or how much energy you are expending, or whether any of these things change. He doesn't even know whether you are taking your insulin properly.

The proper management of diabetes really means sorting out the relationship of three things: your food intake; your insulin dosage and timing; and your energy expenditure. If you can get this relationship right you should be able to achieve your ideal weight and keep it there; do as much work as you need, or want, to; keep your blood sugar levels within safe limits so as to avoid danger and long-term complications; and lead an entirely normal life. That is the ultimate aim of diabetic control, and that is what this book is all about.

All three factors, food intake, insulin and energy expenditure, have an immediate effect on the blood sugar, as you have seen. Food intake raises the blood sugar; insulin and physical work lower it. So, first, diet.

The importance of diet

We have seen that some mild diabetics can be 'cured' by diet alone. In these cases, the purpose of the dieting is simply to lose weight so that the limited insulin supply will suffice. In

41

the case of the insulin-dependent diabetic, diet is even more important. Every mouthful affects the blood sugar level and the control of this level is the responsibility of the person concerned.

You will already have been given excellent dietary instructions, tailored to your personal requirements and taking into account such factors as your insulin dosage, your ethnic group and previous eating habits, your weight, your age, your job, your sporting habits and so on. On these factors, your proper daily calorie intake will be calculated and the prescribed diet will probably be arranged to get you gradually to your ideal weight.

Modern dietary ideas for diabetics are a great improvement on the old and take into account the effect of diet on general health, quite apart from diabetes. For instance, the former emphasis on cutting down on carbohydrates had the effect of forcing diabetics to concentrate on proteins and fats, with dire consequences, especially in men, to their hearts and blood vessels. The new recommendations emphasise the importance of a high carbohydrate diet, with high fibre content, and reduced fat and protein. Nowadays, it is usually recommended that at least 50 per cent of the calorie intake is in the form of carbohydrates. But a high-carbohydrate intake does *not* mean lots of sweet things. You can usefully think of carbohydrates as falling into three groups:

Class of Carbohydrate	*Effect on blood sugar*
1 Sugar, sweets, sweet foods	Immediate rise
2 Starch foods, like bread and potatoes	Intermediate rise
3 Starch in vegetables	Slow rise

By high-carbohydrate intake I mean a high proportion, in the diet, of groups 2 and 3, and practically *no* intake of group 1 (unless required in hypoglycaemia). What we are trying to avoid is sudden peaks of blood sugar and this is exactly what group 1 carbohydrates will cause. Obviously, the carbohydrate intake must be spread fairly evenly over the day and a good way to do this is to divide the total carbohydrate intake into four. You can then take one of these fourths at each of the three main meals and spread the remaining fourth over the gaps, as snacks between meals.

Probably the best way of sorting out your carbohydrate intake is the '10 gram exchange' system, and this is extensively used. Your ideal daily calorie intake will have been worked out, on the basis of the factors mentioned above, and about 50 per cent of your calorie intake will be carbohydrate. It is easy for the dietitian to work out how many grams of carbohydrate this involves, and, by dividing this figure by ten, to get the number of 'exchanges' you can have each day. When you know this figure you can look up a table of 'exchanges' and see what you can safely eat.

Calories (total)	Number of exchanges Carbohydrate (grams) (to provide 50% of cals)	Exchanges (no. of)
2000	240	24
2300	270	27
2400	280	28
2500	300	30
2600	320	32
2700	330	33
2800	330	33
2900	340	34
3000	350	35
3200	380	38
3400	400	40
3600	420	42
4000	450	45

Looking firstly at the *number* of exchanges you are not expected to follow this table with mathematical precision.

You will see that the table makes no distinction between 2700 and 2800 calories. But, used in conjunction with a table of 'exchanges' (see below), it will provide you with an excellent guide to safe carbohydrate intake, while still allowing good variety in your diet. Suppose, for instance, that you are a fairly active girl of 18. You will probably be told that your daily calorie requirement is 2300. Fifty per cent of this will be taken in carbohydrate, that is 1150 calories, and this will be provided by about 270 grams. So you will have 27 'exchanges' to choose from. But if you are a very active labouring man requiring 3600 calories a day, you must take about 420 grams of carbohydrate, which is 42 'exchanges'.

In order to give you plenty of variety, tables of exchanges are quite long, and I have included one at the end of this chapter, but here is a short and especially healthy one which concentrates on carbohydrates with high-fibre content.

High-fibre exchanges	
All-Bran	3 level tablespoons (tbsp)
apple	1 normal size
baked beans	2 level tbsp
broad beans	2 level tbsp
butter beans	2 level tbsp
damsons	10 (stewed)
figs	1 (stewed)
peanuts, salted	100 gram packet
peas, fresh	4 heaped tbsp
peas, tinned	2 heaped tbsp
plums	3 large
prunes	4 medium (stewed)
porridge	4 level tbsp (cooked)
puffed wheat	4 level tbsp
raspberries	6 level tbsp
Ryvita	1 biscuit
Shredded Wheat	1 portion
Vitawheat	2 biscuits
Weetabix	1 portion
wholemeal bread	1 small slice

Each of the quantities on the right is one exchange so, in the unlikely event of a lumberjack, who loves baked beans, wishing to take his entire carbohydrate intake in this form, he could have a total of 90 level tablespoons of beans in the day.

Fats and proteins

So far as these are concerned, the remaining 50 per cent of the calories are divided between them. The usual ratio would be about one-third protein and two-thirds fats, but this may vary a good deal, in the direction of more protein and less fat, depending on personal preference and whether weight is to be gained or lost. When there is temporary increased energy expenditure it is best to make up for it by an increase in the fat and protein part of the diet. Should there be a permanent increase or decrease in energy expenditure the whole calorie requirement should be revised and this is a matter for the diabetic clinic.

Insulin in control of blood sugar

We are aiming to keep the blood sugar levels between 3.5 and 8. Don't worry about the units – they are 'millimoles per litre' but it is quite correct just to think of them simply as figures indicating the amount of sugar in the blood. It is impracticable to imitate the body's normal response to a blood glucose rise. The healthy pancreas might send out a shoal of insulin molecules ten or twenty times a day in response to meals, snacks, consumption of sweets, glasses of beer, cups of sugared tea, and so on, and we could hardly expect to be able to match all these rises. A masochistic diabetic who actually enjoyed giving himself many injections a day, and who was also an expert at calculating the calorie value of everything that passed his lips, could no doubt maintain excellent control of his blood sugar.

But most people find two injections a day quite enough, so we must see how best to manage to control the four main peaks of blood sugar (after breakfast, lunch, supper and the bedtime snack) with only two injections. A common way to do this is to use two different kinds of insulin, together, in each injection – a quick-acting insulin mixed in the syringe with a medium-acting insulin. This has two advantages. It allows a rapid but prolonged effect and it allows considerable flexibility by permitting adjustment of the dose of each of the types.

With a new diabetic, the doctor really has very little idea, at first, what dosage of insulin will be required and has to make an intelligent guess to start things going. The response will soon show how well he has estimated.

Let us see what happened to Michael. After recovering from his diabetic coma and having his fluid situation and ketosis sorted out, it was decided to start him on a diet which would build up his weight to normal. To control the blood sugar resulting from this he was prescribed twice-daily injections of a mixture of soluble insulin (Actrapid) and medium-acting insulin (Retard) and, now that he was up and about and living a normal active life, this was to be taken in a dosage of 12 units of each, at each injection.

Michael was shown how to do the 'Clinitest' method of measuring the level of sugar in his urine (see Glossary for details). By this method he was able to find out whether his urine contained any sugar, and, if so, how much. Here is the Clinitest range:

Negative ¼ ½ ¾ 1 2 over 2 per cent.

He was told that he was to test his urine just before each of the four meals and it was carefully explained to him that he was not to test urine which had been secreted some time before, but was to empty his bladder half an hour before producing the new sample for each test. He was to consider the range from ¼ per cent to 1 per cent, inclusive, as acceptable, but that action was required if he got a negative result or a result of 2 per cent or over. And the action was to change the dose of insulin he was taking, going up by 2 units if the sugar was over the acceptable range and down by 2 units if a negative result occurred. Michael became quite interested in this business and, using the charts that he had been given, kept neat records, on one line for each day, showing the date, the four insulin doses and the four urine sugar readings.

Michael was told that the first Actrapid dose – taken, with the Retard insulin, before breakfast – would cover his breakfast sugar rise; the first Retard dose, being delayed in its effect, would cover the lunchtime rise; the second Actrapid dose, taken before dinner along with the Retard, would act quickly to cover the dinner rise; and the second Retard dose would deal with the supper rise. So he watched each of the four urine results and adjusted the dose of the appropriate insulin, according to the result. His doctor, knowing that most diabetics need between 40 and 80 units a day, had guessed fairly correctly and Michael did not have to change the dosage very much.

He also developed a clear picture of the effects that unusual exercise and being late for meals had on the urine sugar and discovered that the stress of exams, too, could raise the level. He soon learned that he should not change his insulin dosage for purely short-term effects, the causes of which were clear, but that he could deal with those by minor adjustment of his diet.

Measurement of blood sugar

Michael's quickness to learn, and intelligent grasp of the principles, pleased his doctor and he always found time to answer Michael's questions.

'What I would really like to know,' said Michael one day, 'is the actual levels of glucose in my blood. The urine tests are a bit crude, aren't they? I mean, they only tell me that the blood sugar's going too high. Isn't there some way of actually measuring the sugar levels?'

'Certainly,' said the doctor. 'Would you like to monitor your blood glucose?'

'That would be great,' said Michael. 'I think I have a pretty good idea of how and why it varies but I would really like to check directly to see if I'm right.'

'Good,' said the doctor. 'Then we'll go ahead.'

'More needles?' asked Michael.

'Just one drop of blood. We can let you have a gadget that bleeds you fairly painlessly and you will need a supply of Dextrostix and a Glucochek pocket meter.'

Michael was delighted with this extension to his scope for monitoring. The equipment he now had enabled him to measure the blood sugar levels with an accuracy of plus or minus 1 millimole per litre, and he was now able to gain increasing insight into the effects of all sorts of influences and to adjust his food intake and exercise to keep the levels within the acceptable range. The pricker was a spring-loaded gadget that struck his thumb so fast that he hardly felt anything. One drop of blood was put on to the Dextro-stix strip and left for exactly one minute – there was even a timer on the meter – and was then washed off before the strip was put into the meter. The Glucochek meter was the size of a pocket calculator and had a digital readout.

'I don't want you to be too hasty about changing your insulin dosage,' said the doctor. 'You certainly shouldn't change it on the basis of a single high blood sugar reading. That might be due to a sort of rebound that often happens from hypoglycaemia——'

'The Somogyi effect?'

The doctor looked surprised. 'That's right!' he said. 'It's got to do with adrenaline and other hormones, forcing your liver to shoot out more glucose. This happens most often at night and if that's giving you a high blood sugar reading, you would need less insulin, not more. Do you understand?'

'Sure,' said Michael. 'I've read about the Somogyi effect ... So I'm to ignore a single high, and if the levels come down again, I don't change anything.'

'Right,' said the doctor. 'Don't change the dose until you've had highs for four or five days and, even then, change only one insulin at a time. But, naturally, if you get other signs of insulin insufficiency——'

'Like thirst and peeing too much——?'

'Exactly! Then you would put up the dose of one or both of your insulins.'

'I get it,' said Michael.

Glycosylated haemoglobin

'I know you like long words,' said the doctor, 'so I have another one for you. I expect you've heard of haemoglobin——'

'Of course,' said Michael. 'It's the stuff in the red blood cells that carries oxygen——'

'Right. Well, some of the haemoglobin in the red cells – between 6 and 8.5 per cent, to be precise – combines with glucose to form stuff called "glycosylated haemoglobin". The level of this in the blood gives us a really useful measure of the sort of average blood sugar levels over the previous two months or so. People who have been poorly controlled have higher levels than normal. It's a real give-away. I've actually had patients bring me a neat record of normal blood sugars, but with no prick marks on their fingers and a markedly raised glycosylated haemoglobin——'

'Big Brother is watching you!' said Michael.

The doctor smiled. 'Exactly!' he said. 'You're not going to get away with it!'

'Only an idiot would want to!'

'You'll be all right,' said the doctor.

Summary of blood sugar control

- Decide on calorie needs, based on way of life
- Take at least half your calories in carbohydrate (medium and slow release). Remainder in protein and fat. Fast-release carbohydrate only in hypo emergency
- Use 10 gram equivalents for carbohydrates
- Divide carbohydrate intake into four parts and take in four meals, or three meals and snacks.
- Don't miss the bed-time snack
- Master the art of urine testing, but always test RECENT urine
- Your doctor will prescribe insulin or tablets and decide dosage and timing, but YOU will be the one to check that these are correct
- See if you can get into blood glucose testing – this is the best way of all

List of 10 gram exchanges

Each of the following weights of food contains 10 grams of carbohydrate:

Food	Weight/volume
banana	55grams
beer	1pint
Bournvita	15 grams
chappati	15 grams
cherries (with stones)	120 grams
cider	½ pint
Coca-Cola	100 ml
cocoa powder	15 grams
cornflakes	15 grams
cream crackers	15 grams
currants	15 grams
dates (with stones)	20 grams
drinking chocolate	15 grams
flour	15 grams
grapes	60 grams
greengages (with stones)	120 grams
Horlicks	15 grams
ice cream	60 grams
jelly	60 grams
lager	1 pint
milk	200 grams
nectarines (with stones)	90 grams
orange squash	30ml
oranges	120 grams
Ovaltine	15 grams
parsnips	90 grams
pasta	15 grams
pears (raw)	120 grams
peas (fresh or frozen)	120 grams
peas (tinned)	60 grams
pineapple juice (unsweetened)	90 grams
plain biscuits	15 grams
potato chips	30 grams
potato crisps	25 grams

Food	Weight/volume
potatoes (boiled)	60 grams
potatoes (roast)	45 grams
rice (boiled)	30 grams
Rice Krispies	15 grams
Ryvita	15 grams
shortcrust pastry	20 grams
spaghetti (raw)	15 grams
spaghetti (tinned)	85 grams
stout	300 ml
strawberries	180 grams
sultanas	15 grams
sweet corn	45 grams
tangerines	120 grams
white bread	20 grams
yoghurt (fruit)	60 grams
yoghurt (plain)	180 grams

6 PRACTICAL POINTS

When to inject insulin

We have seen that insulin is always given before meals and, as time must be allowed for the absorption of the insulin, this makes sense. But how long before? The standard advice given by most doctors is 30 minutes, but the matter is not usually emphasised and many patients report that they were just told to take the insulin before meals. So, partly for reasons of convenience and partly because of a fear of hypoglycaemia, many diabetics take insulin only 15 or 20 minutes before the meal. Some habitually take their insulin even nearer to the time of the meal.

Medical trials done in Cambridge under the auspices of the Medical Research Council have now shown that, up to a limit of 45 minutes, the longer the interval between the injection and the start of the meal, the better the control of blood sugar and the less the risk of hypoglycaemia. U100 insulin is more concentrated than 40 or 80 unit insulin and is absorbed even more slowly. This makes the longer interval even more important. So the best advice is that you should organise your routine so that you can give yourself the injections not less than 30 minutes before the appropriate meal. If you are doing your own blood glucose monitoring you may be interested to try extending this to 45 minutes.

Insulin strengths

For many years, British and European diabetics have had to put up with a confusing system of syringe marking using two strengths of insulin – 40 units per ml and 80 units per ml. The syringes have 20 marks to the ml, so, if you are using 40 unit insulin, each mark gives you 2 units, and if you are using 80 unit insulin, each mark gives you 4 units. This, in principle, is simple enough to most people, but when you then have to do mental arithmetic to work out how many marks you need to give you the required dose, the chances of error increase.

Happily, for most diabetics, this system is a thing of the past. In 1983, the British Diabetic Association managed to bring about the change to a single-strength insulin of 100 units per ml. Now there are no sums to be done in the head and each mark on the syringe means one unit. You MUST, of course, use U100 syringes. These have the official title of BS 1619/2. Another bonus is that because the insulin is stronger, the amount to be injected is less. Someone taking 20 units of 40 unit insulin used to have to inject half a ml. Now they inject only one fifth of a ml (20 marks). Well over 80 per cent of British diabetics are now using U100 insulins and this brings them into line with American, Canadian, Australian and New Zealand diabetics who have had the sense to use the U100 system for years.

Glass syringes or plastic disposables?

Glass syringes have an average life of about six months and work out a good deal cheaper, in the long run, than plastic disposable syringes and needles used once and thrown away. For this reason, only glass syringes are, at present, routinely available on the NHS. Most people prefer the plastic disposables because they are lighter, unbreakable and don't need to be kept in special containers, but you can have these only if 'they are considered medically essential for a particular diabetic patient'. Pressure is, however, being brought to bear on the DHSS to allow disposables and some authorities have suggested that they are just as safe as glass syringes, even if used repeatedly. In the meantime, some patients find them so much more convenient than glass syringes that they are willing to buy them.

Glass syringes, with the needle attached, should be kept in the container provided and this should be half filled with normal industrial methylated spirit, not surgical spirit. Surgical spirit contains an oily ingredient which makes it unsuitable. The syringe should be taken apart once a week and, together with the container, thoroughly washed with warm water and washing-up liquid. Be sure to dry the metal parts carefully to avoid rusting. After drying, half fill the container with meths and put the syringe with its needle back in the spirit. That is all that is necessary. The syringe need not be boiled.

How to draw up insulin

The secret is to inject some air into the bottle before withdrawing the piston of the syringe. If you don't do this, the removal of fluid leaves a partial vacuum in the bottle so that it gets harder and harder to get the solution out. Get into the habit of injecting a slightly larger volume of air than the volume of fluid to be removed and you will have no trouble. Don't inject too much air or you may waste insulin by having it squirt out when you remove the needle. Be careful that the needle point doesn't touch anything hard – it is easily blunted and this will make injections more painful.

You will probably be mixing two insulins in the same syringe – a rapid- and a medium- or long-acting insulin. This means two different bottles and you will not be able to inject air into the second one once you have drawn up insulin from the first. So the secret is first to inject air into the second bottle, then pull out the needle and inject and withdraw insulin from the first bottle. Then push the needle into the bottle already pressurised and withdraw the required amount. Avoid getting any long-acting insulin into the bottle of fast-acting insulin or it will no longer be rapid and this could cause trouble. With a little practice you should become skilled at holding the bottle and the barrel of the syringe in the same hand, leaving the other to withdraw the piston. But if you find this difficult, keep the syringe pointing straight upwards and the needle will easily take the weight of the bottle.

How to perform the injection

You should not inject successively in the same place as this may make the area hard and lumpy from fibrous tissue formation and, worse still, may lead to uncertain absorption from the site. There are plenty of places to choose from and you should move from one to the next in a strict routine. Use the upper and outer parts of the arms and of the thighs, the outer parts of the buttocks and anywhere on the abdomen. Assuming your skin is clean and dry, no skin preparation is necessary. If you are thin, you may have to pinch up the skin. If fat, stretch it. Check that the needle is firm on the syringe so that it will not come off while you are injecting. Never touch the metal part of the needle as you will contaminate it and may possibly carry germs deep under your skin and cause infection. In fact, this is very uncommon, so long as your standards of cleanliness are reasonable.

Insert the needle with a quick jab, vertically into the skin, almost as if you were throwing a dart. Do not go in at an angle, as you may then inject too near the surface. Don't draw back the piston before injecting insulin. If the needle is in a blood vessel the insulin will simply be absorbed a little more rapidly than normal. Inject slowly, wait for a few seconds, then pull the needle out quickly. If there is bleeding, press with a dry cotton ball for a minute or two. Don't worry about isolated bruises. They will absorb in two weeks. If you bruise frequently, tell your doctor and he will check whether your blood-clotting system is working properly.

Urine testing

The level of blood sugar at which glucose 'spills over' into the urine varies quite a lot from person to person but is, on average, about 10. So if the urine test shows 0.25 per cent or more, the blood sugar level, at the time the urine was secreted, is likely to be 10 or above. Don't forget that a casual urine test for sugar does *not* tell you the state of the blood sugar at the time of the test, because the urine you are testing may have been produced by your kidneys quite some time before. This is why it is important to empty your bladder, then wait until you can produce a little more fresh urine for the test. Even then, the result, as an indication of the blood sugar, will be somewhat out of date and it might, of course, be falsified by the presence of some older urine, if you did not completely empty your bladder.

There are many different ways in which the urine can be tested and you would do well to stick to the method you are accustomed to. If you use Clinitest tablets remember to close the bottle tightly as these tablets soon deteriorate if exposed to the air. Remember also that they contain corrosive chemicals (caustic soda and copper sulphate) and would cause serious injury if swallowed. So keep the bottle firmly closed and out of reach of small children.

Clinistix and Glucotest strips are simpler and less trouble to use. Diastix are also very convenient, but if there are lots of ketones in the urine, the acidity will spoil the test and may even give you a negative result when sugar is present. So you must also be interested in the possible presence of ketone bodies and should test for these, especially if there is more than 1 per cent of sugar in your urine. Ketostix will detect ketones and Ketodiastix will detect both. Because diabetes can affect your kidneys (see Ch. 12), you should also be on the lookout for albumin. Albustix will reveal albumin. In all cases you must follow the instructions carefully and note especially the importance of timing. A timer with an alarm signal is a useful and not very expensive accessory.

How often should urine be tested?

If you are insulin-dependent you should test your urine for sugar four times a day – before each of the four meals. Always write down the result. Be wary if the result remains constantly negative because you are at risk from hypoglycaemia. Tell your doctor. Tell him also if the figure remains steadily above 1 per cent. Tell him whenever you detect ketone bodies.

If you are on diet only, or diet plus tablets, test your urine at least once a day and always do it about two hours after the largest meal of the day. Your urine should always be free of sugar. If you find sugar, test your urine four times a day before meals. If sugar persists, tell your doctor.

What to do if you are sick

Any sort of major illness, or any illness lasting for more than three days, is definitely a matter for your doctor. But what about colds, influenza, tummy upsets and other minor or short-term illness? These, too, can sometimes be quite important, especially if there is vomiting or diarrhoea, and the latter should *always* be reported to your doctor. Vomiting and/or diarrhoea can quickly reduce the proper levels of fluid in your body and this can be serious for you.

The next thing to remember is that you should modify your normal routine as little as possible. You may not feel like eating but you should try to maintain the normal intake if you can, and balance it with the normal dosage of insulin. If you find you can't take your normal food, try to replace it with liquid carbohydrates like fruit juices, milk shakes, jellies or even fizzy drinks. Half a cup of orange juice or ginger ale is one 10 gram equivalent.

Never omit an insulin injection for fear of a hypo. Test your urine at least four times a day, for both sugar and ketones. Always drink plenty of fluids. This is especially important if there is abnormal fluid loss, as from sweating, vomiting or diarrhoea. If you are taking much more than the usual amount of fluid, keep a record of the amounts drunk. Watch out for the carbohydrate content of the fluid drunk.

If you are in any doubt – consult your doctor.

Effects of other medical treatment?

This is important and you should be clearly aware of the way in which drug treatment can affect the results of your urine testing. The most important drugs are aspirin and vitamin C. Ordinary headache doses will not have much effect and can be ignored, but if, for any reason, you are taking more than 8 tablets a day your urine will contain enough acid to affect the result. Many people take large doses of vitamin C and this appears in the urine and can affect the tests. A few of the other drugs which can have this effect are Aldomet (methyldopa), Levodopa, Benemid, Ceporin (Cephalosporin antibiotic) and Nalidixic acid. Because of the duplication chaos over drug names you might be taking some of these without knowing it; therefore, if you are on any long-term treatment at all, check (tactfully) with your doctor that he has remembered this possibility.

All diabetics are, or should be, extremely sensitive to the sweetness of anything taken by mouth. But you may not think there is any harm in taking necessary medication by mouth, even if this tastes sweet. Unfortunately, some medicines contain a considerable quantity of sugar and you must watch out for things like cough mixtures, linctuses, elixirs, medicinal syrups, antibiotic suspensions and so on. These could give you an unexpected glucose boost and cause changes in the urine test results.

7 HYPOGLYCAEMIA

In Chapter 1 we saw how uncontrolled diabetes can eventually lead to the production of high levels of ketone bodies and coma. But there is another, and quite different, way in which coma can occur in diabetes and that is what this chapter is all about. In diabetic coma the blood sugar level is very high. In hypoglycaemic coma it is very low. This never happens on its own and cannot happen in diabetics treated by diet. It can happen only in people treated with insulin or tablets.

The distinction between these two conditions – excessively high and excessively low blood sugar – is of central importance and no diabetic can afford to be confused about it. Hypoglycaemia is a dangerous condition. Why? Because the brain must, at all costs and at all times, have an adequate supply of glucose. Unlike the muscles and the liver, the brain doesn't have its own glycogen storage system. Thus, any shortfall in the supply will have rapid, widespread, and sometimes devastating, effects.

'Hypo-' means 'under, below, less than', '-glyc-' means 'glucose' and '-aemia' means 'blood'. So the word simply means 'not enough glucose in the blood' or 'low blood sugar'. It is essential that not only diabetics, but also, as we shall shortly see, the members of their families, should know all about it – what causes it, what it does, what are its symptoms and effects and how it should be treated. Hypoglycaemia can occur in a number of ways. Let me tell you another story.

Mandy, a twenty-two-year-old insulin-dependent diabetic, believed in leading a full life and was an enthusiastic cyclist, who went to work in Westminster every day on her bike. She was reasonably careful about her insulin and diet and had not had a great deal of trouble with her control. For weeks she had been looking forward to the Brighton cycle run and had been cycling fast each morning to tone up her leg muscles in preparation for the event. The great day dawned and she was up early. After taking her usual 60 units of Semilente insulin and her usual breakfast, she set off on her bike to Clapham Common for the start of the run.

It was a lovely late June day, slightly overcast, perfect cycling weather, and Mandy felt on top of the world. Her brother Neil was waiting at the rendezvous they had agreed on and they clocked through the departure channel a little before nine. With a 56-mile run before them, they sensibly decided to take it easy. Neither of them were anxious to make a race of it. By the time they had reached Redhill, soon after eleven, the sun was fiercer and they began to feel rather hot. Mandy began to sweat.

'D'you think we'll make it, Neil?' she asked.

Neil looked at her in surprise. She looked quite anxious. 'What d'you mean, "make it"?' he said, scornfully. 'Of course we will!' Then, in a more kindly tone, 'Are you all right? You look a bit pale.'

'Of course I'm all right. Come on!' Mandy forged ahead.

Not long after that they came to a major road crossing manned by police and traffic wardens. The cycle traffic was heavy and cars were piling up on either side. A policeman waved them through but Mandy cycled up to him and stopped.

'Keep moving, Miss!'

Mandy got off her bike and laid it down in the middle of the road.

'Come on, Mandy!' said Neil, embarrassed.

Mandy went up close to the policeman and pulled his cap down over his eyes. Her hands were trembling and when she spoke her voice was slurred and shaky. 'That's the wrong way!' she said.

The policeman pushed back his cap and said, good-humouredly, 'No larks, now Miss! On your way!'

Scores of cyclists were riding past the scene, watching curiously. Mandy put her arms round the policeman's neck and slumped on to his chest. Another policeman came up.

'Need any help, Bert?'

'This one's zonked. Can you get her off of me?'

The second policeman pulled Mandy away. She looked as if she were only half-conscious. Her hands and arms were twitching and her face was making curious grimacing and sucking movements. The two policemen carried her to the side of the road and laid her down on the verge. Neil picked up Mandy's bicycle and wheeled the two machines off the road. He parked them and went to her.

'She's my sister,' he said.

'Well, you should look after her,' said one of the policemen. 'What's she on?'

Neil was getting alarmed. 'What do you mean?' he asked.

'Doesn't smell of drink . . .' said the first policemen.

The penny dropped. 'Oh God!' said Neil. 'It's her diabetes! She's having an attack! It must be that! She needs insulin!' Frantically, he fumbled open the bag on Mandy's bicycle and got out the syringe kit.

'Hold on!' said the policeman. 'Do you understand about this?'

'Not really,' said Neil. 'But she takes insulin.'

'Well,' said the policeman. 'I don't think we should give her any. She could be having a "hypo"——'

'What's that?' asked Neil, frantically. 'We must do something!'

'There's an ambulance and a doctor at the next checkpoint,' said the policeman. 'Come on!'

Ten minutes later, by courtesy of a concerned motorist, the comatose Mandy was lying in an ambulance being attended to by a young white-coated doctor.

'She takes insulin, does she?'

'Yes,' said Neil.

'Do you know how much?'

'No. Sorry.'

'I suppose she had it this morning?'

'Sorry, I don't know. She has her own flat in Streatham.'

'Did she have breakfast?'

'I don't know. Probably.'

'No question of drugs, glue, anything like that?'

'No. Mandy's a fitness freak. She's not interested . . .'

The doctor had been sniffing Mandy's breath. She was now deeply unconscious and completely relaxed. He came to a decision. Taking a vial of 50 per cent Dextrose solution and a large disposable syringe and needle, he drew up a syringe-full and put a tight rubber tube round Mandy's arm. 'Hold that,' he said.

'What are you doing?' asked Neil.

'Giving her sugar.'

'Sugar! Hasn't she got too much already? She needs insulin, doesn't she?'

The doctor compressed his lips, but said nothing. When the needle was in the vein, he asked Neil to release the tourniquet. The sugar solution was given slowly, directly into Mandy's blood-stream and within a few minutes, to Neil's intense relief and surprise, her eyes fluttered open.

Mandy's recovery was complete and, in spite of having been in coma for twenty minutes, she suffered no discernible brain damage. But the episode taught both her and her brother a much-needed lesson and Neil now saw that his ignorance of even the basics of her condition had been unpardonable. The doctor had taken Neil aside just before Mandy was driven off to hospital. 'Insulin would have killed her,' he had said.

How to recognise a hypo

There are several important lessons to be learned from this story. Mandy took her usual insulin dose before breakfast, and the amount she ate was appropriate to that dose. By the time she reached Clapham her blood sugar had reached a reasonable level and everything was satisfactory. But during the next two hours Mandy expended far more than her usual amount of energy and soon used up, to fuel her hard-working leg muscles, not only the sugar provided by her breakfast but also the glycogen stored in her liver. When she asked Neil if he thought they would make it to Brighton she was displaying the typical anxiety reaction of early hypoglycaemia. Had she been more experienced, she would have recognised this, and the tremor of her hands that went with it, as a hypo effect, and would have sucked a couple of glucose sweets. This would have been sufficient to prevent all the subsequent unpleasantness.

What caused the feeling of anxiety? You remember that low blood sugar causes a release of adrenaline into the blood for the purpose of forcing the liver to give up its glucose rapidly and to get cracking with the manufacture of new glucose (gluconeogenesis). It is this adrenaline that caused the feeling of anxiety – some people experience real panic – the tremor of the hands, the fast pulse, and so on. As Mandy's blood sugar dropped further, her brain began to be deprived of its essential fuel (this happens when blood sugar drops below about 2). The brain can no more function without a constant fuel supply than can a car, and as soon as the brain function falters, the effects are obvious. Mandy's behaviour with the policeman was irrational and quite out of character and was due to failing function of the higher, and most sensitive, parts of the brain – the parts that are affected first by alcohol. Soon, the effect on Mandy's brain was more widespread and the part controlling the muscles of her face was affected, causing the twitching and sucking movements. Finally, the deeper parts were knocked out and she lost consciousness.

I want to emphasise that the symptoms of hypoglycaemia vary from person to person and also depend, to some extent, on the rapidity with which the blood sugar falls. But, for any particular individual under similar conditions, the effects are reasonably constant and should be readily recognisable. Remember that the initial effects are caused by adrenaline, the 'fright, fight and flight' hormone, and that symptoms then arise from brain malfunction. In these, the most advanced functions of the brain, such as judgement, are involved first. So the first brain effect is usually odd and uncharacteristic behaviour.

There is one exception to this which, fortunately, is quite

rare. Some people with long-standing, poorly controlled diabetes may develop a form of diabetic neuropathy (see Ch. 12) involving the brain, which deprives them of the ability to recognise the signs of hypoglycaemia. Such people, who are usually elderly, may become unconscious from low blood sugar, without any warning.

Here is a fairly full list of the kind of things that can happen in hypoglycaemia:

	Hypoglycaemia
Adrenaline effects	*Brain fuel deprivation effects*
Worry	Hunger
Rapid pulse	Skin over-sensitivity
Sweating	Shakiness
'Sinking feeling'	Double vision
Nausea	Sense of unreality
Pallor	'Drunken' behaviour
Belching	Yawning and tiredness
Rapid breathing	Unsteadiness
	Weakness
	Lightheadedness
	Muscle twiching
	Regular muscle spasms
	Fits
	Loss of consciousness
	Abnormal deviation of the eyes
	Enlarged pupils
	Deep coma
	Shallow breathing
	Slowing of the pulse
	Death

The causes of hypoglycaemia

By now, you are probably able to work out most of these for yourself, but they are so extremely important that I am going to list them for you:

- Too much insulin
- Insufficient calorie intake, eg. missed meals
- Excessive exercise in relation to calorie intake
- Illness, especially infection
- Drugs (see below)
- Alcohol liver damage and other liver diseases (see below)

There are some rare causes of hypoglycaemia, such as tumours that secrete insulin, but these need not concern us.

Is hypoglycaemia always so severe?

No. The picture I have painted is the picture of a severe 'hypo' occurring rapidly. Some people on long-acting insulin, whose dosage is too high, have less obvious effects and tend to show the brain deprivation signs rather than the adrenaline signs. So they may seem to have developed a change of personality with lowered standards, apparent laziness, deterioration in work performance, loss of memory and irrational behaviour. Such people are often thought to be drunk or drugged. All these effects may result from chronic (long-lasting) hypoglycaemia, either from insulin or sulphonylurea overdosage or from inadequate carbohydrate intake. It can also happen if a diabetic deliberately takes less food than is required.

Genuine alcoholism, in conjunction with diabetes, is a deadly combination as the liver damage plays havoc both with the vital glycogen store mechanism and with gluconeogenesis.

Hypoglycaemia during sleep

The possibility of this happening often causes diabetics great concern. Many fear that they will go into coma and never wake up. Happily, this is almost unheard of, but lesser degrees of hypoglycaemic effects during sleep are quite common. Again, the danger is more likely with people using long-acting insulin, as this may actually have its maximum effect after the person has gone to sleep. If this is worrying you, here are one or two signs which may give you a clue to whether this is happening:

- Disturbed sleep
- Nightmares
- Sleeping in unusual positions
- Crying out during sleep
- Sleepwalking
- Bed-wetting
- Headache on waking

The new occurrence of any of these should alert you to the possibility and you should report them to your doctor. Some modification of insulin dosage, or type, may be necessary, or it may be sufficient just to increase the size of your late-night snack a little.

The Somogyi effect

Night-time hypoglycaemia may occasionally have another effect, which was first described in 1953 by a man called Somogyi. The low blood sugar can prompt a large production of the anti-insulin hormones glucagon, adrenaline and cortisol. These, in turn, force your liver to release a considerable quantity of glucose, and you may wake up with a great deal of sugar, and even ketones, in your urine. This is a dangerously misleading situation as you may think you need more insulin when, in fact, you need less. If you suspect that this is happening, or if you are worried, in general, about night-time hypoglycaemia, the best thing to do is to set your alarm for the middle of the night and monitor your blood sugar.

This hormone-induced rise in blood sugar, in response to hypoglycaemia, may sometimes even occur during the day, so bear the possibility in mind if you find unexpected things happening.

The urine in hypoglycaemia

Many people are confused to find that, during a hypoglycaemic attack, the urine may show the presence of sugar. It is important that you should be clear about this and not allow it to mislead you. During a 'hypo' the blood sugar is low and the urine secreted contains *no* sugar. But of course, if you give a sample of urine which your kidneys produced some considerable time before – at a time when your blood sugar was high – and which has been stored in your bladder, this urine may contain sugar. But if you now empty your bladder and then, a little later, test a sample, it will be clear. Even doctors have occasionally been led astray by this effect, but you, knowing the timing of events, should never be misled.

Drugs which can cause hypoglycaemia

If you are being treated for high blood pressure or heart trouble with 'Beta blocker' drugs, you could have problems. These drugs reduce the effect of adrenaline which, as we have seen, is a powerful sugar-raising hormone. So they can cause a drop in the blood glucose. Note, also, that because of the 'blockade', you will not experience, to such a marked degree, those hypo symptoms caused by adrenaline (see above, p. 00).

There is a group of drugs used for the treatment of depression and anxiety called the 'monoamine oxidase inhibitors'. These include Elamol, Marplan, Nardil, Niamid and Parnate and they all have some effect in increasing the action of both insulin and diabetes tablets. So, although they are unlikely to do so to such an extent as to cause hypoglycaemia, they might just occasionally be the cause of an otherwise unexplained hypo. Quite a number of other drugs can have a similar potentiating effect, but only on the sulphonylurea anti-diabetic drugs. These include Atromid-S (which is sometimes used to treat diabetic retinopathy), Chloromycetin, Aureomycin, Terramycin and, of course, the Sulphonamides.

None of these is likely to cause serious interference with the treatment of your diabetes, but it is as well that you should be aware of the risk.

8 CHILDREN AND DIABETES

If you are the parent of a diabetic child you will already have gone through the shock and distress – perhaps even the feeling of panic-struck helplessness – that assails those who, without any special qualification, suddenly find themselves placed in a position of responsibility for the health and even the life of a loved one. It is not a pleasant experience, but you will, by now, have got over the worst of it and will already have learned enough about diabetes to realise that the responsibility is not beyond you. I would like, in this chapter, to do what I can to lighten that burden of responsibility. The disease processes of diabetes, and the principles of management, are exactly the same in children as in insulin-dependent adults and most of what I have told you in this book will be relevant. A careful study of these principles is, therefore, basic to your management of your child's case.

But the diabetic child undeniably presents special problems and this is not simply because someone other than the patient must take on the job of maintaining control. In the adult patient, body growth will have ceased so that the nutritional requirements are fairly stable. But the diabetic child is growing and developing and requires every bit as much food intake as any other child of the same age. So there will be constantly changing requirements of diet and insulin dosage – another fact which makes it imperative that you should understand the principles. Diabetic children always need insulin, but usually quite a small amount is sufficient and in a great many cases a single daily dose is all that is needed. This is fortunate because, at the beginning, the injections may be an ordeal both for the child and for

68

you. You may be assured, however, that this stage will pass very quickly and that it will not be long before the child will be able to give the injections himself. This should be encouraged as early as possible, but, of course, careful supervision is important to ensure that everything is being done properly. Particular attention must be paid to the care with which the correct dosage is drawn up and given.

The young diabetic child will seldom be able to describe symptoms or to give you any real help in deciding whether the present dosage of insulin is correct or whether there is a risk of hypoglycaemia. But, although an awareness of symptoms may be very helpful in adult diabetics, as an indication of their own condition, you will always be able, even without this assistance, to judge the state of the child. A constant awareness of the urine sugar levels, a sensitivity to the signs – rather than the symptoms – of hypoglycaemia, an unobtrusive but regular watch over the child's general behaviour and state of activity and, if necessary, even a check of the actual blood sugar – all these will tell you how things are going.

Young diabetic children cannot be expected to show responsibility over their own diet and they always have to be disciplined. Prohibition of sweets is something a young child takes very hard and you may find it particularly difficult to deny the child what seems to be an indication of your affection. Fortunately, a child's perception of your love is not measured in terms of sweets and, if everything in your relationship with the child is as it should be, he or she will, without really understanding why, accept the prohibition as a necessary part of the misfortune of being a diabetic.

One of the strongest instincts in children is to conform to the patterns of behaviour set by their friends, and the diabetic child is at once recognised as 'someone different' – not only in the restriction in what he or she may eat, but also in the necessity to have regular injections and fairly close supervision. This sense of being different may produce a feeling of alienation and increase the child's resentment at the apparent denial of pleasures freely available to friends. So, as a parent, your responsibility is not only heavy, but sometimes painful, and great courage and patience will be required of you to ensure that, within the limits of safety, your child lives as normal, full and happy a life as possible.

This responsibility is too great to be borne by the mother alone, as, regrettably, seems often to be the case, and fathers must realise that the burden on a mother of young children is already very great without the additional concern over trying to understand diabetes and to carry out the necessary management. The greatest part of this additional burden is mental and concerns the awareness that the child's life may, almost literally, be in one's own hands. Only knowledge and understanding of the nature and effects of diabetes can relieve this stressful anxiety and it is here that the caring father can do much to help. The father of a diabetic child, who, instead of accepting the primary responsibility, leaves the whole management to his wife and does not even take the trouble to understand the disease, is behaving in an irresponsibly selfish manner. Such a father must not be surprised if he finds the mother giving more attention to the diabetic child than to him.

So the first requirement is for both parents to understand the fundamentals of diabetes. Everything you need to know can be found in this book. Study the subject together, discuss it, learn the meaning of the terms, argue over it, get to be experts, vie with each other in acquiring expertise. As your knowledge grows, your fears will fade.

A normal life for your child

As I have repeatedly emphasised, elsewhere, the object of the modern management of diabetes is to maintain normal health with the minimum of interference with the life of the subject. Indeed, it is now clear that, for the maintenance of full health, a diabetic must, in addition to ensuring good blood sugar control, lead an active life with plenty of vigorous exercise and a good balanced diet. This must be your aim for your growing child and it is not an aim which can always easily be achieved. It means, for instance, that, unless you are willing and able to participate in your child's sports and games, you may have to accept a measure of worry as you delegate to others the supervision over these activities. Walking, jogging, swimming, climbing and, for the more affluent, skiing and other winter sports, should ideally be a family affair, with no discrimination made between the diabetic and other children. These activities are often very popular with children and adolescents, and little urging may be necessary to encourage participation. But some young people are naturally sedentary and these may have to be pushed a little. A healthy interest in competitive sports can be an excellent thing for the young diabetic.

A high level of energy expenditure on strenuous activity is an excellent thing for the growing diabetic child and you should be thoroughly familiar with the effect of such exercise on the blood sugar and the insulin needs so that you will be able to adjust the insulin dosage as required. It should be perfectly plain to you that if a young person is stabilised on a particular diet and insulin dosage, and if that person then increases the average amount of exercise taken – say, by regular cycling, football, athletics, gymnastics, dancing, etc. – the amount of insulin needed will become less, perhaps quite a lot less. But remember, also, that the effect on the insulin requirement works both ways. Should the child, for any reason, have a sudden drop in the energy expenditure, the blood sugar, and the insulin need, will rise. This will, of course, be reflected in the appearance of increased sugar in the urine, so conscientious urine checking is especially important at times of change in the activity levels.

How much can be left to the child?

In the case of the young child, of course, nothing. For very young diabetics, everything must be done, and that is the period when a trustful relationship is developed between the child and both parents, so that proper habits and attitudes are formed and accepted. But as the child grows and enlarges his experience of the world, two things will happen. On the one hand, he will become aware of his difference from others of his own age and will begin to question his parents' rule. On the other, the child will, through the desire to achieve growing independence, be forced to accept that he must do more and more for himself and that will include giving himself his own injections and checking his own urine for sugar.

This stage is not without its own dangers. Remember how strong the temptations may be for the young person to yield to the impulses to be exactly like others – especially in the matter of food and sweet things – and face the possibility that your child may not be beyond cheating in order to get his or her way. There are plenty of cases on record of young people falsifying their urine test records in order to conceal the fact that their carbohydrate intake is much higher than it should be. Children have deliberately diluted their urine to give a low sugar reading, or even borrowed urine from a brother or friend. To those of us who understand the implications and dangers of such practices, it may seem extraordinary that a young person could be so foolish. But it is essential for us to remember how powerfully young people can be addicted to sweet things and how almost irresistible may be the craving in those deprived.

In many cases this problem has been so serious that it has been found better to allow a small ration of sweets and to cover this with additional insulin, rather than to run the risk of occasional secret binges. Some children take very badly to a total prohibition and feel justified in cheating. This is a point on which you must make up your own mind. A small regular ration of sweets – perhaps 20 grams – taken following meals, and especially in the form of 'diabetic sweets' (which allow what seem to be a larger quantity for the same calorie value, but which, unfortunately, are really just proportionately less satisfying) may be preferable, in some cases, to total prohibition. Saccharin is sometimes acceptable to children, but this should not be used unless the craving for sweetness is very strong. Not that there is any special danger in the use of saccharin – it's just that it is better to try to get the child accustomed to a generally unsweet diet – which is, in any case, an altogether healthier state of affairs for all of us.

72

If other children in the family are allowed sweets, the sense of injustice may be acute and this is a point you will have to decide upon. Much consolation can be afforded the diabetic child by allowing moderate quantities of low-carbohydrate fruits such as blackcurrants, gooseberries, loganberries or melon, as extras to the normal diet. Remember, also, that the child may feel less discriminated against if some of the 10 gram equivalents are given in unusual form – perhaps to the diabetic child only – such as peanuts (120 grams per 10 gram exchange), chestnuts (30 grams), almonds (230 grams) or dried raisins or sultanas (15 grams per exchange).

Young people have been known to omit insulin, perhaps out of dislike of injections, but more often as a protest against authority. The effect of this will, of course, soon become apparent and the child will become ill, with high urine sugar levels and perhaps ketoacidosis. Even in the absence of these signs, this may well be a problem you should not try to handle on your own. And, of course, if your child does become ill from this cause, medical attention, perhaps admission to hospital, will be necessary. The effect of this will be to impress on the child the seriousness of what he or she has done and may prove the solution to the problem.

Sometimes children will simply refuse to eat, and parents may be driven to distraction. But remember that carbohydrate exchanges can very easily be given in the form of a drink, and a child will often take liquid when solid food is refused. Check your tables of 10 gram exchanges and try to tempt the rebel with milk shakes or fizzy drinks.

It is essential for the growing child progressively to take on responsibility for his or her own control and health and this responsibility must be based on clear understanding of the principles. It is your duty, as a parent, to ensure that these principles are understood. Having achieved this, you must then place a good deal of trust in the young person. But this trust must be realistically tempered with suspicion based on a clear awareness of the stresses and temptations to which your child is exposed.

Diet

The growing child requires a considerable calorie intake, for fuel must be supplied both for current energy expenditure and for promoting growth. Active children – and children *should* be active – may have a calorie requirement almost as great as that of a sedentary adult, so it is important to ensure that worry over blood sugar does not lead to undue restriction on intake. An average child of five will probably need about 100 grams of carbohydrate each day and this will rise to about 160 grams daily by the age of ten and about 200 grams per day by the age of fourteen. Remember that the carbohydrate must be divided between the main meals and the snacks (see Ch. 5) and that carbohydrate should be selected from the 'slow release' groups. These figures are, of course, only average and children and adolescents who can be encouraged to engage in regular strenuous exercise may well need more. After puberty, there will tend to be greater variations in the energy expenditure.

But even more important than ensuring an adequate calorie intake, is the necessity to ensure that your child does not establish habits of excessive food intake. Any amount of food can, of course, be covered by insulin, but to use this fact to allow excessive intake and the development of early obesity, is a major disaster which will have life-long repercussions. This pattern is especially likely to occur if you, the parent, are prone to excessive food intake and obesity, for you will probably have a special emotional reaction to food and will tend, almost instinctively, to want to feed your child in the manner that you yourself were fed as a child.

Children who are made fat by parental over-indulgence are likely to find it difficult or impossible to control their weight throughout life. There is a physical reason for this and it is as well that you should be aware of it if you are not to expose your child to a considerable social and health disadvantage. When adults of normal weight settle down to a physically less active life but continue to eat as much, they become overweight, laying down fat around the middle of the body – the tummy, waist and buttocks, but almost never on the shoulders, back and extremities. This extra fat is simply filling up existing fat cells so that they are stretched. No new fat cells are produced. But when obesity occurs in childhood, there is a fundamental difference in that an actual, and considerable, increase in the *number* of the fat cells occurs. And this increased number of fat cells – distributed about the body – persists throughout life and makes it 'natural' for such people to eat much more than is good for them.

If you are obese, the probability is that your mother, misguidedly, although doubtless with the most loving intentions, got you, at an early age, into the wrong shape and pattern of eating habits. So it is now up to you to break the cycle.

Education

As the diabetic child grows, education becomes progressively more important. Your child will begin to learn about diabetes from the moment the disease starts and he discovers that he is to have regular injections. He will accept the necessity without understanding it, as he will accept the necessity for dietary restrictions, and these things are part of his education. But as the child grows in understanding, mere unthinking acceptance is not enough, and you should make it your business to ensure that, at the earliest reasonable stage, he or she begins to be taught the reasons for this strange discrimination. Training – in urine testing, in blood-sugar testing, in the recognition of hypoglycaemia, in diet control and in the proper way to give injections – can all be achieved early; but as soon as possible the child should be made to understand about the function and effects of insulin, about the relationship of blood sugar to diet and exercise, and about the way in which alterations in these things call for alteration in insulin dosage.

By early adolescence, a reasonably bright boy or girl should be able to make his or her own adjustments to food intake and insulin dosage, so as to cope with varying levels of energy usage and even to handle the effects of minor illness. The adolescent who quickly reaches this level of understanding will develop a great interest in the subject and will be proud of his or her mastery of it. Those, on the other hand, who have not been given adequate instruction will be frightened and increasingly resentful, and serious problems, both medical and social, are likely to arise.

Above all, adolescent diabetics must be schooled in the central importance of good control as a means of avoiding future complications. Intelligent young diabetics, sometimes convinced that they know much more about the subject than their doctors (and occasionally they do!), will sometimes resent the time wasted hanging about diabetic clinics and will default from attendance. It is no good trying to frighten these young people into submission by horror stories of blindness and kidney failure. What is important is to make sure they understand that avoidance of these and other complications is possible and that proper medical check-ups can give early warning of trouble and provide a chance of treatment. Adolescents require a higher standard of medical care than any other group of diabetics and deserve the best that is available.

The saddest thing of all is to see young adults present with serious and sometimes irremediable complications who might, with good advice and caring guidance, have been spared them.

9 DIABETES AND DAILY LIFE

You have probably felt, from time to time, that it is a little unreasonable for doctors to tell you that you should lead a normal life when, at the same time, you are expected to cope, almost entirely on your own, with a disease that affects almost every aspect of it. People with other major chronic diseases are not expected to monitor their own progress and treat themselves, and large concessions are usually made to them. It's all very unfair. But that's the way it is with diabetes and it isn't going to do you any good to feel sorry for yourself. Diabetes is very bad luck, but the world is full of admirable people, in every walk of life, who, in spite of it, manage to live not only normal lives but useful, gratifying and productive lives.

You want a few examples? How about Paul Cézanne, H.G. Wells, Thomas Edison, Spencer Tracy, Jack Benny, Mary Tyler Moore and Harry Secombe? Many successful athletes and sportsmen and women have been insulin-dependent diabetics and have managed to maintain good control in spite of the increased problems caused by the heavy energy expenditure. Examples are Billie Jean King the Wimbledon Champion, Gary Maddutt the English footballer, the Olympic walker Mike Holmes, David Croft the skater, and British golfers Mark Lye and Elizabeth Price.

Exercise and sport

So one way in which you can aim to live fully is to determine to keep your muscles and your heart–lung system in first-class order. This demands exercise – not just the occasional

77

burst of activity, but a determined, sustained policy of regular daily physical work: walking instead of driving, using stairs instead of lifts, regular jogging, deliberately getting a little breathless at least once a day. Such a course, unless already habitual, will necessarily require a change in your dietary/insulin pattern – more calories and less insulin. But beware of a sudden increase in exertion. Work up to it gradually, adjusting your intake of food and insulin, on medical advice, as you go, and then keep it up. Always carry glucose. Regular daily exercise should be enjoyed by everyone and there is no reason why diabetics should be left out. Indeed, if you use your diabetes as an excuse for avoiding health-bringing exercise, you are breaking a basic rule.

If you are a professional or keen amateur sportsman you will be aware that you require special management, for it is impossible for you to maintain the relatively even levels of sugar production and expenditure which are the ideal for the less athletic diabetic. Since you must engage in short periods of intense physical activity, in which you will use up fuel at a tremendous rate, there will be considerable variations in your insulin requirement and you may have to cut down considerably on your insulin dosage before a game or a major race. Some professional footballers use up blood glucose at such a rate that they have to cut their insulin dose to a quarter of their normal intake on the day of a match, or they experience hypoglycaemia.

Diabetes by no means precludes professional sport, but you will need expert advice and assistance both at the preliminary stage of rebuilding muscle bulk and once you are back on form. You will, of course, never think of starting a match without glucose tablets or sugar lumps in the pocket of your shorts!

Employment

So far as the risks from hypoglycaemia are concerned, this is simply a matter of common sense, and responsibility rests entirely with you. You have to consider not only your own advantage and the risks to your own safety, but those of others. If you are prone to hypo attacks you would be crazy to take a job cleaning the outside of the top windows of the Millbank Tower. Driving buses and heavy goods vehicles is also not for you. Although modern factory machinery is now much safer, the safeguards do not necessarily legislate for someone liable to hypo attacks, and exposure to such risks may be best avoided. The Armed Services have entry rules which exclude insulin-dependent diabetics, but do not necessarily discharge those who develop diabetes during service. If you are thoroughly familiar with the early signs of hypoglycaemia and can react appropriately, you will probably feel that you are safe to drive a car. The matter is one for your own conscience.

Surveys have shown that – dangerous occupations apart – diabetes, in itself, has little or no bearing on a person's suitability for employment. Individual physical or mental capacity, education and experience are what counts. The disease itself is largely irrelevant. Some diabetics will use their condition as the reason for their inability to hold down a good job, but the unfortunate people who do that would probably have another explanation for their failure if they were not diabetics. The great majority of diabetics, however, like the great majority of people generally, do a job entirely in accordance with their ability.

Regrettably, these facts are not always recognised by prospective employers, and highly suitable candidates are sometimes turned down when it is learned that they are diabetics, usually on the grounds that they are likely to be frequently off work on account of the condition. Again, a survey, undertaken by the British Diabetic Association, has shown that this is a misconception and that diabetics lose less time from work on account of diabetes than the generality of workers do on account of other medical conditions.

Travel

If you don't normally carry a card, or wear a bracelet, indicating that you are a diabetic (and you certainly ought to), this is one thing you must see to before you set out on your travels. Indeed, if you are going abroad it is a good idea to carry with you, in addition, a medical certificate confirming the diagnosis and outlining your treatment. This could prove handy in the unlikely event of questions being asked about your syringes at customs posts. Ask your doctor to write down the official (generic) name of your insulins, as the local name in the overseas location is likely to be different. But, in any case, be sure to take plenty with you.

When flying, always tell a hostess that you are diabetic, ask for a diabetic diet and indicate when you need to eat. This is especially important when crossing time zones. Never travel, in any case, without some source of sugar, as you may still encounter delay in serving your meals. Carry your insulin and syringes in your hand baggage, not in the hold baggage – which might end up anywhere. Try to keep the insulin bottles reasonably cool, but don't panic about this as insulin is reasonably stable and will maintain its potency for a month or two, even at temperatures up to 25°C.

Ignore any announced time changes and leave your watch set at home time. Carry on with your normal insulin and dietary routine for the whole of the journey and be especially careful about urine testing. At the end of your journey, local time will be earlier or later than your personal time. If you have travelled westward your watch will be ahead of local time so you will have some extra time to cover and will need additional insulin, in proportion to the amount of time to be made up. Of course, if you have gone half round the world, you will be able to continue your insulin at the normal intervals, but a six-hour gain will call for a supplement before you can reset your watch. Always be guided by the urine result or, better still, by your blood glucose measurements. On the way back, travelling eastwards, you will lose time and will need less insulin.

If you are travelling on holiday, watch out for any major change in the amount of your activity. Some change is likely as you will not be following your normal way of life. The thing may go either way and you should be prepared to make the appropriate adjustments. You should not plunge into frantic winter sporting activity if your way of life is normally sedentary; no one should, of course, without a proper preliminary work-up to full physical fitness – but a diabetic who skips this stage risks more than just orthopaedic problems.

Sex

Because quite a lot of men with diabetic neuropathy (see Ch. 12) have suffered organic impotence, the view has got about that diabetes is likely to interfere with your sex life. This is, of course, nonsense. There are plenty of causes of sexual disturbance but organic interference from diabetes comes low on the list. There are, however, one or two ways in which diabetes can indirectly influence your chances of long-term sexual contentment and these are worth mentioning.

Women diabetics are more prone to vaginal thrush (candidiasis) than non-diabetics, and this condition can cause local irritation and even pain during intercourse. Both partners may suffer symptoms. Symptoms of this kind should not be ignored, but should be freely discussed and reported to your doctor. Proper gynaecological investigation and treatment with one of the modern fungicides can always put this condition right. Your partner should also be treated.

Some doctors have advised against the use of the IUD (intra-uterine contraceptive device) because of the slightly increased risk of infection as a result of minor mechanical injury to the uterus, but this opinion is arguable. The risk seems to be small. So far as the contraceptive pill is concerned, the earlier types – with high oestrogen content – did have a definite effect on diabetic control, but the more recent – and generally safer – low-oestrogen pill can be regarded as fairly safe. You may need some minor adjustment to your insulin dosage.

There is very little reason why diabetics should not enjoy a full and satisfying sexual life. Women, in particular, need have few problems. But diabetic men will still tend to worry about their potency and, of course, such worry is one of the commonest causes of psychological impotence. In this way a vicious circle can easily be induced, in which the man, observing a falling-off in his sexual powers, attributes this to early diabetic neuropathy and suffers further failure from increased worry. A man in this situation may not be much helped by reassurance, for his doctor will have to admit that it is not very easy to distinguish between organic impotence from diabetic neuropathy and psychological impotence.

To add to the problem, poor diabetic control can cause temporary loss of male sexual capacity and this, too, may be interpreted as neuropathy. Happily, with restoration of good diabetic control, and in the absence of a major psychological problem, the sexual powers will return. The difficulty is to avoid the effect of anxiety about potency. Relaxation, a rejection of 'macho' values, mutual acceptance, a sensitive and loving partner and a clear understanding of the nature of psychological impotence will do much to resolve this problem. The majority of diabetic men with potency problems do not have neuropathy.

A number of diabetic men have had vasectomies out of an exaggerated idea of their chances of producing a diabetic baby. This is not, in itself, a good reason for taking such a step, for the chance is small – about one in a hundred.

Diabetes and other illnesses

You have to remember that almost any other illness or injury, or even major mental stress, is bound to affect your diabetes so that you need more insulin. This applies, also, to surgical operations. Why is this? Your body reacts to all these things by producing hormones – steroids, growth hormone and adrenaline – all of which act against insulin and favour release of sugar and fats into the blood. The extent to which these hormones operate depends, of course, on the severity of the stress-producing event. If you were involved in a major road accident, even if you were not badly injured, this would certainly have a striking effect, at least for a time, on your diabetic control. Major injury would have a greater and more prolonged effect. Infections affect you in exactly the same way and you must be aware of the risk and realise that you have two problems to deal with.

So, however well-controlled and stable your diabetes may be, you have to expect that injury or illness of any kind will upset your control. You must watch your urine results, or better still, your blood glucose levels, most carefully. Be especially on the lookout for ketone bodies in the urine and report this to your doctor without delay. Vomiting is a bad sign and may indicate the urgent need for an increase in your insulin dosage. Your doctor may well, temporarily, change your present scheme of dosage for repeated injections of quick-acting insulin.

If you need a surgical operation, you will probably be admitted to hospital two or three days before, so that your control can be stabilised and you can be checked over for complications of diabetes. The anaesthetist will be especially careful to avoid hypoglycaemia and it is likely that you will go to theatre with a drip of dextrose solution running. Insulin can be added to the drip so that everything can be kept under perfect control.

10 STAYING HEALTHY

To stay healthy must be the central aim of every diabetic, and I hope it isn't necessary, at this stage, to remind you that full control over your blood sugar is basic to the issue. The loss of health in diabetes really means the development of diabetic complications. Non-diabetics – whose blood sugar is automatically kept normal – don't get diabetic complications; so, if you want to avoid them, you must see to it that your blood sugar levels are kept as nearly as possible within normal limits.

But staying healthy doesn't just mean avoiding disease. Health is a positive, dynamic thing, which should be associated with a feeling of well-being. And you will not get it by lying on your shoulder-blades in an armchair, drinking beer, smoking cigarettes and watching TV. Smoking is a pernicious enough habit for the non-diabetic, for the diabetic it is disastrous. I'm not thinking of the small but real risk of lung cancer, but of the very much greater risk of damage to your blood vessels and heart, which, with the additional risk of angiopathy, makes smoking almost criminal. There are much pleasanter ways for diabetics to commit suicide than by smoking. Don't even consider it!

Regular vigorous exercise should be a central feature of your life and, as I have already explained, your insulin should be adjusted accordingly. Walk, whenever you can, instead of driving; take up a sport and play every week. You can play golf at any age and walk for miles, chasing the ball, without noticing. It goes without saying that your diet should be satisfactory. At least 50 per cent of your calorie intake should be carbohydrate – and slow-release, high-fibre carbohydrate at that.

Alcohol

Like everything else in the diabetic dietary, alcohol must be treated with caution and taken in moderation. Since the aim is to lead a full and pleasant life, it would be a pity to deny oneself this notable aid to social intercourse. But one or two points must be made. Alcohol can interfere with the release of sugar from glycogen in the liver and so may cause hypoglycaemia. This possibility makes drinking and driving a particular hazard for diabetics, which should always be avoided.

Don't forget, either, the high-calorie value of spirits – 7 calories per ml of pure alcohol. This is almost twice the calorie value of sugar. To save you mental arithmetic, this means that there are 100 calories in every 50 ml (2 fl oz) of whisky or gin. Beers and lagers, on the other hand, being more dilute, push up the calories rather more slowly. You can have a pint of beer or lager, or a half of stout or cider, as one 10 gram carbohydrate exchange. If you fancy diabetic lager, you can really make a splash – 2½ pints for one 10 gram exchange.

Severe over-indulgence in alcohol is another major disaster for the diabetic. You now know what an essential part normal liver function plays in the storage and release of glucose, and you can easily see how dangerous it could be if that function were disturbed. Alcoholic cirrhosis of the liver will do exactly that.

Attitude

A healthy, realistic attitude to your diabetes is important. You can never know too much about the condition – including all the unpleasant features. There is simply no point in burying your head in the sand. Much better to know about these things and see to it that they never happen to you. The best way to keep from being morbid about your diabetes is to live actively, strenuously and positively, determining to emulate the many distinguished diabetics who, in spite of their disease, manage to do more with their lives than many who are spared the disease.

But, in addition to all that, there are some other matters that should especially concern you, particularly if you are elderly or have had the misfortune already to suffer some complications. Some are simply the application of common sense, but it will do no harm to mention them.

Looking after your skin

Remember that you are more prone to infection than other people, and don't forget that *candida* is very fond of sugar. Jennifer suffered 'down below', but the same fungus can also attack your skin elsewhere, causing an itchy, red, oozing area surrounded by small pus spots. This is most likely to affect areas where there is skin-to-skin contact and you may really have problems if you are very fat and there is constant, moist rubbing between your skin surfaces. The combination of warmth, moisture, sugar and minor skin damage from friction is likely to prove irresistible to the thrush fungus. Avoid tight clothes, such as jeans, or unnecessarily tight underwear. Cotton is better than most man-made fibres for clothing next to your skin.

Candida albicans is not the only fungus likely to attack uncontrolled diabetics more enthusiastically than other people. There is another nasty one called Trichophyton which, with one or two close associates, can attack any part of the skin, but especially the groin and feet, to cause the various types of itchy 'tinea' or, as it is popularly and inaccurately called, 'ringworm'. 'Athlete's foot' is one of these. The same fungus can get under the fingernails and toenails to cause a particularly unpleasant and persistent infection which can lead to softening and crumbling of the nails. Fortunately, there is a drug, Griseofulvin, which can deal effectively with these creeping nuisances.

Other infections may be troublesome, especially pimples, styes, boils and even carbuncles (multi-headed boils). A crop of such infections should alert you to the possibility that your blood sugar control may be slipping, and you should always report such events to your doctor.

You may notice yellowish, flat areas in the skin, especially around your eyelids or over bony points, such as the elbows. These are deposits of fats and may indicate that your blood cholesterol levels are too high. Take note of the warning and act on it. Point these out to your doctor and ask him to investigate their implications.

Another form of fat deposit, but this time underneath the skin, may form if you get into the bad habit of always injecting in the same place. I appreciate that you want to do this because of the lesser discomfort of using an insensitive area, but this practice will lead to the formation of fibrous tissue (deep scarring) and this will interfere with the absorption of the insulin. You may, as a result, be having to take unnecessarily high doses, so that enough gets through to the blood-stream in time. It may also affect the accuracy of control. So do rotate the injection sites as you have been instructed. If you have scars where you have been injecting, you are probably not going deep enough. Inject perpendicularly – not at an angle.

Check regularly for oedema of the skin (fluid collection) especially around your ankles and feet and in front of your shins. Press on the skin with your thumb and see if a slowly filling hollow is left behind. This is an important sign which should always be reported to your doctor. It could be an indication of kidney trouble.

Finally, be on the lookout for painless injuries such as burns. It is not uncommon for diabetics with neuropathy to let cigarettes burn down between their fingers, so that the skin becomes scorched and blackened, without their being aware that anything untoward is happening. Inspect your hands regularly and never ignore such injuries.

The feet in diabetes

Problems with feet are very common in diabetes and if you are an older, insulin-dependent diabetic, you must be aware of the dangers and understand how to avoid them. Let me remind you that these dangers come from three causes:

- Nerve damage
- Reduction in blood supply
- Infection

Diabetic nerve damage can, as we have seen, cause widely differing effects. One of these is to reduce the sensitivity of feeling in your skin so that minor damage can occur without your being aware of it. Because your feet are exposed to mechanical injury of various kinds, and because even minor injury can lead to more serious things, you are especially liable to trouble if you don't look after them properly.

Because blood carries the vital oxygen and nutrients, all the tissues of the body require a good blood supply for health. Unfortunately, as you should now be clearly aware, diabetes can damage blood-vessels and lead to a reduction in the local blood supply. This may, occasionally, be so severe that local areas of tissue – even entire toes – are entirely deprived of blood and simply die. This is called gangrene and is, of course, extremely serious. But even short of that stage, a partial reduction in blood supply can reduce the efficiency of healing and encourage infection.

Infection is especially likely to occur if injured areas are neglected, and many a serious foot complication has started with quite minor damage, such as may occur from careless cutting of toenails. When these three factors – nerve damage, poor blood supply and infection – operate together, you are likely to have trouble. But there are certain rules which, if observed, may greatly reduce the risk of what might become a serious complication, and you should note these carefully and always stick to them.

How to look after your feet

- Make sure your shoes fit properly. They must not be too tight. When new, break them in gradually. Don't wear very high heels which force your toes against the tip. Don't wear open-toed or open-heeled shoes. These can cause pressure sores.

- Check your shoes for internal roughness, foreign bodies, etc. If your fingers are not very sensitive, get someone else to do it for you. Corns are an indication that your shoes do not fit well. They can be dangerous. DO NOT CUT CORNS. Get the chiropodist to attend to them.
- Don't wear stockings or socks with holes in them and don't wear darned stockings. When holes occur – throw them away. Wear clean socks each day.
- Wash your feet every day and dry them thoroughly but gently, especially between the toes. Treat the skin with respect. After washing, inspect them carefully looking for any signs of skin damage, especially ulcers and blisters.
- Cut your toenails after washing and don't risk cutting down into the corners of the nails. Just cut straight across.
- Keep your feet warm, especially at night. Wear bed-socks if your feet feel cold. Don't risk hot water bottles. You may not realise that you are being burned.
- Don't wear garters or even very tight clothes, such as jeans. These can compress blood vessels and interfere with the blood supply to tissues that are already at risk. They could tip the balance in favour of severe complications, even gangrene.
- Above all, don't ignore damage to your feet, however unimportant it may, at first, seem. Report it to your doctor without delay so that it can be attended to and complications may therefore be prevented.

11 PREGNANCY

I'm afraid this chapter is going to cause anxiety, perhaps distress. If you are already pregnant, or are contemplating pregnancy, you will not find much comfort in it. But the message is not so much one of gloom as of warning and positive advice, so that everything possible can be done to eliminate or minimise the dangers, both to you and to your baby. Millions of diabetic women have gone through pregnancy uneventfully and happily and have produced normal healthy babies. But you are going to have to face the fact that, as a diabetic, you are more likely than non-diabetic women to have trouble. So this chapter is terribly important for you, and you should read every word with care.

Much depends on the severity of your diabetes. As you will read below, there are women with complicated diabetes who should, quite definitely, avoid pregnancy altogether. There are also some with severe and poorly controlled diabetes, who might find it difficult to conceive and, in these cases, this is probably just as well. But for the general run of diabetic woman it is only too easy to get pregnant. Note that it is only because of *your* diabetes that problems are likely to arise. If your husband is diabetic and you are not, then you have nothing to worry about, so far as the pregnancy is concerned.

It is an unfortunate fact that pregnancy has a tendency to make diabetes worse or to bring to light diabetes that had previously been unsuspected. If you are mildly diabetic, you will almost certainly need more insulin during pregnancy, but, after delivery, will probably return to your former requirements. The trouble is that the hormones which are produced in large quantities during pregnancy, especially by the placenta, have a definite anti-insulin effect. In women who are established diabetics, this will lead to a greater insulin requirement, but it may also actually cause diabetes in those who were previously apparently healthy. Unfortunately, the effect is not always temporary and sometimes persists after the baby is born.

If you are not diabetic, you should be wary if any of the following factors apply to you:

- A family history of diabetes
- Excessive weight
- A previous delivery of an unusually heavy baby
- A previous stillbirth

These are hints that you may be at risk of developing diabetes during pregnancy, and you should not fail to mention this to your doctor, who will arrange appropriate tests.

Diabetes and the stages of pregnancy

There are seldom any great problems during the first three months of pregnancy – indeed, during this period, diabetic mothers-to-be quite often need less insulin than usual. But once the first three months are past, things tend to get difficult and the need for increased insulin dosage becomes obvious. Very careful control is essential because of the changing situation and insulin dosage will usually have to be increased substantially. High maternal blood sugar levels and ketone bodies are dangerous to the baby, and both may readily occur in pregnancy.

Just to make matters even more complicated, pregnant women often suffer a lowering of the levels at which their kidneys allow sugar to 'spill over' into the urine. This lowered 'renal threshold' causes real problems and means that monitoring of the blood sugar situation, by urine testing, may be misleading. Fortunately, the growing availability of reliable, portable equipment to monitor the blood sugar levels directly is helping to overcome this difficulty. The lowered threshold for sugar also has the undesirable effect that a great deal of glucose can be lost in the urine. So, a careful diet and insulin dosage, calculated on the basis of the usual assumptions, may go astray. Sometimes there is even significant interference with nutrition.

For these reasons it is advisable for pregnant diabetic women to be admitted to hospital on the first signs of loss of stabilisation and, since problems tend to be at their worst in the last three or four weeks of the pregnancy, it is common to bring about delivery, either by inducing labour or by doing a Caesarian section, at about the 36- or 37-week stage. In spite of the early delivery, babies of diabetic mothers are often larger and heavier than normal. They should always be checked by a paediatrician very soon after birth. A drop in the baby's blood sugar is common during the first few days (see below).

The effect on the baby

The mother's insulin doesn't get to the baby, but the mother's raised blood sugar does. This forces the baby's pancreas to pour out insulin and, as a result, the baby turns the excess sugar into fat and muscle and, especially towards term, the rate of growth is abnormally high. This is why babies of diabetic mothers are often overweight at birth. But when the baby is born, it is immediately deprived of the extra sugar supply and, because it may still be producing excess insulin, there may be hypoglycaemia.

Malformations in babies born to diabetic mothers are about three times as common as in babies born to non-diabetic women, and there is clear evidence that the probability of such misfortune increases if diabetic control is poor. These malformations include heart abnormalities, spina bifida, neurological defects and abnormalities of the skeleton. Sometimes these malformations cause stillbirth, but, tragically, death of the baby sometimes occurs, late in pregnancy, even with an apparently normal baby. Severe ketosis in the mother is very dangerous to the baby – about a 50 per cent baby mortality.

I mentioned glycosylated haemoglobin in Chapter 5 and

explained that this was a valuable way of checking, retro-spectively, on the standard of control. The upper acceptable limit seems to be 8.5 per cent and a trial in 1981, based on this figure, drew some very sobering conclusions. The study was done on 116 diabetic pregnant women and the levels of glycosylated haemoglobin were checked in early preg-nancy. Of those with less than 8.5 per cent glycosylated haemoglobin, 3.4 per cent had babies with abnormalities. In the group with more than 8.5 per cent, no less than 22.4 per cent produced babies with major deformities.

All the indications are that this is simply due to high sugar levels in the very early weeks of pregnancy and it seems clear that, if such tragedies are to be avoided, it is too late to start thinking about diabetic control once conception has occurred. It has been recommended that young women at risk should be advised at a 'pre-pregnancy' clinic where contraception and the importance of diabetic control can be discussed. When pregnancy occurs the baby should be examined by the method of ultrasonic scanning (which is much safer than X-rays) so that major abnormalities may be detected early and, if appropriate, the pregnancy terminated.

Apart from congenital abnormalities, babies of poorly controlled mothers also tend to suffer other early disorders. These include jaundice, excessively thick blood, low blood calcium and the dangerous 'respiratory distress syndrome'. None of these, however, is more common than normal if excellent diabetic control is maintained throughout the pregnancy.

The respiratory distress syndrome

This is a condition, often very serious, in which the lungs of new-born babies are solid, relatively airless and inelastic and cannot pass oxygen on to the blood. It is caused by a deficiency of an essential detergent substance and it was, formerly, very common in the babies of diabetic mothers. The death rate was quite high. Happily, there has now been a major advance, in that a method of detecting lung maturity, before birth, has been developed. This involves taking a sample of the fluid in the uterus – which is done very easily by passing a needle through the abdominal skin – and analysing it for the ratio of two substances produced by the baby. This ratio indicates whether or not the lungs are mature, and whether the baby can be safely delivered. Respiratory distress syndrome is now rare except in very premature babies.

How can good control be achieved?

First of all, education is vital. A young diabetic woman with no idea of the risks of pregnancy will simply carry on as usual. The harm to the baby may even have been done before she knows she is pregnant. So there is much to be said for the idea of 'pre-pregnancy' clinics. It also follows that any diabetic woman who is at risk of becoming pregnant must, at all costs, maintain good diabetic control.

Frequent urine tests are important but remember that pregnancy often lowers the kidneys' 'threshold' for sugar, so these may be misleading. Urine tests are not, however, in themselves sufficient, and pregnant diabetic women should have the blood sugar monitored directly, either in a clinic or by using a portable instrument like the Glucochek pocket meter or the Hypo-count meter. Women who understand the implications are likely to do a more thorough job of monitoring their own blood sugar than is possible in a busy clinic.

The four-dose, two-injection system of insulin dosage is greatly to be preferred for pregnant women than any less flexible form of insulin treatment. Single daily doses of long-acting insulin are not likely to be safe and offer little scope for the careful adjustment of dosage which is so essential during the constantly altering situation in pregnancy. The anti-insulin effect of the hormone from the placenta increases as the pregnancy progresses and it will be necessary to increase the insulin dosage proportionately. In some cases the dose will eventually have to be doubled. Some women will require three injections a day. Those who are unable or unwilling to cooperate in the maintenance of good control should be admitted to hospital.

Complications of pregnancy

Three of the common complications of pregnancy occur more frequently when the mother-to-be is diabetic. These are urinary tract infections, hydramnios and pre-eclamptic toxaemia. I will explain these alarming-sounding names in a moment.

Urinary tract infection is, of course, quite common in any pregnancy, but because the germs which cause infection flourish in the presence of extra sugar, this is especially likely in diabetics – who will usually have sugar in their urine. But although frequent, these infections are not essentially different from other urinary infections and respond well to routine treatment with antibiotics. The case of diabetic women whose kidneys have already been damaged by diabetes (see Ch. 12) is, however, different. Such women are likely to suffer a worsening of the kidney problem. Those women whose kidneys already show obvious signs of diabetic damage ought, very definitely, to avoid pregnancy.

Hydramnios means an excess of water within the womb and this occurs, to some degree, in about one diabetic pregnancy in five. In many cases the condition will be mild and unimportant. A woman with severe hydramnios will seem to be further on in pregnancy than her dates suggest and there is always a risk of premature rupture of the membranes. Happily, there are established ways of dealing with this problem.

Pre-eclamptic toxaemia is the condition in which the blood-pressure rises unduly, fluid collects in the tissues (oedema) and a kidney condition develops which leads to the appearance of albumin in the urine. This trio of signs gives warning of the risk of the much more serious condition of eclampsia in which fits occur and life is endangered. Pre-eclampsia demands the closest ante-natal attention and, if the signs are worsening, the pregnancy must be terminated without delay, either by inducing labour or by Caesarian section.

Effect of pregnancy on diabetic complications

I will deal with the complications of diabetes in the next chapter, but it is important to mention, here, that pregnancy can have such a serious effect on certain established diabetic complications as to justify avoidance or, in some cases, medical abortion. This is especially so with diabetic nephropathy (kidney disease) and certain types of diabetic retinopathy (disease of the retinas). If either of these conditions has already caused obvious trouble, pregnancy should certainly be avoided. And, if the probable alternatives are grave kidney damage or permanent blindness, the question of sterilisation should be seriously considered.

A diabetic woman whose pregnancy results in her being crippled by kidney disease or blinded by internal eye bleeding is going to find it an awesome burden to look after a baby as well as attend to her own diabetes. However much she may want to have a child, a woman with severe and complicated diabetes must be clearly aware of the risk that her own condition may worsen, that the baby may not survive and that, if it does, she may not then be in a position to give it the attention every baby deserves and needs. This is a painful matter, but I think it is entirely proper that such women should be realistically advised so that they are able to make wise decisions.

It would be a pity to end this chapter on such a gloomy note, so let me urge you, if you are a healthy diabetic, to take an optimistic, sensible and balanced view of the whole business. It is important to appreciate that the worst possibilities apply only to severe diabetics with complications. Remember that millions of lovely, normal babies have been born to diabetic mothers, who have been none the worse for their pregnancies.

12 THE COMPLICATIONS OF DIABETES

With this chapter we come to the crux of the matter. It is the presence or absence of the complications of diabetes that make the real difference between a condition which is no more than an annoying nuisance and one which may gravely affect the quality of life or even threaten it. And whether these complications occur or not depends largely on the care with which the diabetes is controlled. Don't let anyone try to persuade you that control doesn't matter.

Take the case of 'old' Mrs MacDonald, who was fifty-three and looked seventy, a widow and an insulin-dependent diabetic for over thirty years. Mrs MacDonald would do a token urine test, every now and then, when she felt a bit seedy and sometimes, when the sugar was 2 per cent plus, she would take 'a wee bit extra' insulin. Quite often she forgot to take any, until the smell of the ketones on her breath reminded her. In spite of what the district nurse kept telling her, Mrs MacDonald didn't really believe that the trouble with her legs had anything to do with her diabetes. 'Sugar dibeets is sugar dibeets,' she would say, with conscious sagacity, 'and cold feet is cold feet.' The nurse had been quite worried about her legs and had tried, regularly, to get her to see her doctor. The skin was very cold and there were two ulcers on the left shin which stubbornly refused to heal. She was unable to feel any pulses, on either side, below the level of the knees.

Surprisingly enough, Mrs MacDonald didn't seem to suffer particularly from the cold. Her feet felt icy, but, although she had plenty of other complaints – especially about her right eye (which had gone blind suddenly, and about which the specialist had said he couldn't do anything) she never complained about any discomfort in her legs. One day, while visiting her to dress the ulcers, the nurse noticed that Mrs MacDonald's little toe, on the left side, had turned black.

'You're for hospital, Mrs Mac!' said the nurse.

'Whit for? There's nothing wrong forby a wee bit discolouration . . . That canna be gangrene! I dinna feel onything.'

But gangrene it was, and the blackening of the toe was quickly followed by an ominous duskiness spreading up the foot. In hospital, the surgical consultant paused at the foot of Mrs MacDonald's bed and the small group of students, who were following him, gathered round.

'Morning, Mrs MacDonald,' he said. 'Don't mind if I talk about you to these young doctors, do you?'

'Talk away, manny,' said Mrs MacDonald, bitterly. 'Tell them why you had to take my leg off.'

'This,' said the consultant, 'is a typical case of peripheral vascular disease, with neuropathy, secondary to diabetes, leading to ischaemia and tissue necrosis——'

'An' what does all that mean, when it's at home?' asked Mrs MacDonald, querulously.

'It means that the arteries supplying your leg with blood got completely clogged up so that the blood couldn't get through. Also, the diabetes had affected the nerves so that the feeling in your feet was defective and you didn't have the normal warning of pain. If you'd had normal sensation, you would have had so much pain that you would have done something about it earlier.'

'Well, I haven't any pain in the other one, either. Does that mean——?'

'We'll do everything we can to prevent that happening, but you must play your part and be a bit more responsible about your diabetes.'

'What's that got to do with it?'

'It's got everything to do with it. Diabetes leads to thickening of the lining of the blood vessels and encourages clotting of blood on the thickened lining. In your case, the clots blocked off the vessels altogether . . .'

He nodded and walked on. When they were out of earshot,

he said, 'Mrs M. is in a bad way. She's quite likely to lose her other leg and she has proliferative diabetic retinopathy which has bled on the right side and blinded that eye. Do you know what proliferative retinopathy is, Gowers?'

A bespectacled student smiled and spoke up. 'Growth of fragile new retinal vessels, sir, usually around the optic disc. Very prone to cause haemorrhage into the vitreous——'

'Good. Treatment?'

'Laser destruction of the peripheral retina, sir.'

'Correct. The ophthalmologists have seen Mrs MacDonald's left eye and confirmed that she has proliferative DR in that one too. They want to laser her, but she's not keen. I expect she'll go blind. What else might she have? Harvey?'

'Nephropathy, sir.'

'Right. What's that?'

'Disease of the kidney, in this case diabetic, with damage to the filtration mechanism and tubules——'

'What does it cause?'

'Protein in the urine, renal failure, oedema, hypertension, secondary pyelonephritis——'

'Correct. Is Mrs Mac likely to have nephropathy?'

'Yes, sir.'

'Why?'

'We know she already has widespread damage to blood vessels – angiopathy – and neuropathy, so it's very likely——'

'Correct. What's the prognosis?'

'Pretty terrible, sir.'

'How long do you give her?'

'Well, I suppose it depends on her future diabetic control . . .'

'Maybe. Probably a bit late for that, now. I wouldn't like to say. But I wouldn't try to sell her any life insurance, either . . .'

What the words mean

I expect you are wondering about all these words ending in '-pathy' – 'neuropathy', 'nephropathy', 'angiopathy', 'retinopathy'. '-pathy', which just means 'disease of', is a very handy ending for doctors who don't want to commit themselves to describing the exact nature of the disorder. In the old days it was '-itis' for nearly everything. 'Neuritis', 'nephritis', 'angiitis', 'retinitis'. But '-itis' means 'inflammation' and most of these conditions are not inflammatory. So the current jargon is less inaccurate, but not really any more revealing.

The four basic major complications of diabetes are:

- Angiopathy – disease of blood vessels
- Retinopathy – disease of the retinas of the eyes
- Nephropathy – disease of the kidneys
- Neuropathy – disease of nerves

Let me deal with these in turn, before dealing with infection and cataract.

Diabetic angiopathy

This links up with retinopathy and nephropathy because the disorders in the retinas and the kidneys are essentially the result of diabetic damage to small blood vessels. But in long-standing, poorly controlled diabetes it is not only the small vessels which are affected. Mrs MacDonald lost her leg because of a condition of larger blood vessels called 'atheroma', and, although this is quite common in older non-diabetics, it occurs much more often and more severely in people like her. In atheroma, plaques of cholesterol and other materials are laid down in the wall of the vessels and these lead to narrowing. Next, there is a tendency for clotting to occur on the part of the inner lining of the blood vessel overlying the plaque, and once such a clot has formed there is a danger that complete blockage may occur. This is called a thrombosis.

Any major blood vessels may be affected in this way and among the commonest to be involved are the coronary arteries, which supply the heart muscle, itself, with blood. Atheroma of the coronary arteries is much commoner in uncontrolled diabetics than in others and so, of course, is coronary thrombosis. Normally, women are much less

100

liable to coronary thrombosis than men, but in severe diabetes they seem to lose much of this relative immunity.

Retinopathy

The retinas are the complex neural membranes at the back of the eyes, on which the images formed by the lens systems fall, and which have the job of converting these images into nerve impulses so that the brain can be supplied with visual information. To work properly, the retinas needs an excellent blood supply, and when diabetes damages their small blood vessels, the retinas themselves are damaged and their function impaired. Damaged blood vessels in the retinas leak both blood and fatty material into the nerve fibres and the resulting tiny haemorrhages and collections of free fat can easily be seen if the retinas are examined with an ophthalmoscope.

This, the milder type of retinopathy, will significantly interfere with vision only if these fatty deposits and haemorrhages occur in the vital central part of the retinas – the parts we use for detailed seeing, such as reading or recognising people. We are remarkably insensitive to loss of peripheral vision, unless it is very extensive, and don't usually notice it. But there is a more severe form of diabetic retinopathy in which the damage to the retinal blood vessels is so severe that the retina decides to do something about it and starts to bud out new blood vessels. You might think that this was a good thing, and no doubt it would be if these new vessels were more strongly made. Unfortunately, they are extremely flimsy and thin-walled and rupture very easily.

This is the essential problem. Diabetic new vessels are an ominous sign because they nearly always bleed profusely, filling the back part of the eye with blood, obscuring vision and encouraging further blinding complications such as fibrosis in the transparent jelly of the eye and detachment of the retina. This is what happened to Mrs MacDonald's right eye, and what was likely to happen to her left also unless she agreed to treatment. People with extensive diabetic new

101

vessels on their retinas, who do not have laser treatment, have about a fifty per cent chance of becoming blind in the affected eye, or eyes, within a year. So it is not a thing to be casual about, and you can understand how important it is to have your eyes regularly checked for this complication.

Nephropathy

The kidneys are remarkable filters, extracting from the blood waste substances like urea, while retaining those, such as protein, fats and sugar, which are required by the body. To do this, great volumes of fluid have to pass through these filters, but, in health, nearly all this fluid is reabsorbed into the blood-stream and only enough is lost to carry away, in solution,the waste material. By causing damage both to the blood vessels of the kidney and to the filtering parts, diabetes can, very gradually, over many years, lead to interference with the normal functioning of the kidneys. Once this has happened, the matter is always serious. Urea can no longer be filtered out of the blood and its levels rise dangerously. At the same time, proteins like albumin, which ought to be retained, escape into the urine.

Diabetes does not, of course, necessarily lead to nephropathy and many diabetics of many years' standing have entirely normal kidney function. But most insulin-dependent diabetics will, after many years, show some signs of kidney involvement, although this is not usually serious. In those who show heavy loss of protein in the urine the outlook is less favourable and many proceed to total kidney failure, at which stage the only hope of survival rests in a kidney transplant. People with severe diabetic nephropathy usually have retinopathy, also, and often have large vessel diabetic disease. This may make the outlook for successful grafting less favourable, as a good blood supply to the grafted donor organ is essential for success.

This rather gloomy account will bring little comfort to those unfortunate enough to have these major diabetic complications, but I hope it may serve as an indication to younger diabetics of the critical importance of good control.

Neuropathy

Nerve damage, in diabetes, involves local injury to the insulating sheath surrounding nerve fibres and, although the fibres themselves may be intact, they are thus made incapable of transmitting the nerve impulses. The legs are most commonly involved so that there is partial or complete loss of sensation in the feet and sometimes in the calves and shins. This is dangerous as the person concerned is unaware of, and naturally neglects, injuries, abrasions, minor infections and so on. These may thus rapidly become worse. Pressure sores and ulcers are common in people with diabetic neuropathy and careful nursing is essential.

Although most of such patients have no pain at all, some suffer acutely painful episodes with persistent aching and burning down the front of the legs. This pain tends to be worst at night when the person is lying quietly.

Neuropathy can affect other parts of the nervous system and can, therefore, lead to a wide variety of effects ranging from interference with normal eye movement, so that double vision occurs, to disturbance of normal bladder function. As we have seen, organic impotence can occur as a result of diabetic neuropathy. In this type of impotence, there is no interference with sexual feeling or desire and the hormonal situation is normal, but the nerves concerned with the control of blood flow to the penis are affected and erection cannot be achieved. Regrettably, there is no effective treatment for genuine organic neuropathic impotence.

Infection

We have already seen that infection is more common and often more serious in diabetics than in other people. Indeed, anyone who suffers frequent recurrences of skin infection, such as boils, or urinary infections, or, for that matter, almost any recurrent infection, should certainly be checked for diabetes. Interestingly, deep tissue infection, which might be expected to be common in people who have to give themselves so many injections, often in a relatively unhygienic way, is remarkably rare. This is a most fortunate circumstance, as diabetics already have quite enough to worry about. But infection is often a major problem in people with neuropathic feet ulcers and, in severe nephropathy, it is often the event which leads to the final kidney failure. Infection, in diabetics, is as susceptible to antibiotic treatment as in anyone else, but should, whenever possible, be reported and treated early.

Cataract

We saw in Chapter 1 how the alteration in blood sugar levels can temporarily affect the focussing of the eyes. Very rarely, this effect can be so severe that the internal lenses become opaque and the person affected may become blind in the course of a few days. This is called true diabetic cataract. It is extremely uncommon and sight can be restored by removing the cataractous lenses, but strong glasses, or contact lenses, will be necessary to restore the focus of the eyes.

Ordinary, old-age cataract occurs in diabetics, as in anyone else, and is in no way different from normal cataract. It does, however, seem often to tend to occur at a somewhat earlier age than usual, but this is hard to be sure about because the age of onset of cataract is so variable. The results of surgical treatment are just as good as with anyone else and, so long as there is no other damage to the eyes, full vision will be restored.

If you are especially concerned about the eye complications of diabetes, you will be able to read more about the subject in another book of mine, *Everything You Need to Know About Your Eyes* (Sheldon Press, 1985) in which I have devoted a whole chapter to the subject.

13 THE FUTURE

This is an age of unprecedented medical advance, and the pessimistic have been proved wrong so often that it would be foolish to say that anything is impossible. But the endless display of new medical wonders makes it even harder for the lay reader to exercise critical judgement as to what is likely to be achieved and what is improbable. So this chapter will be concerned with some of the lines of diabetic research showing promise of being important.

The volume of research in progress on diabetes is enormous and it would be quite impossible to read all the papers being published on the subject. But major advances – or the promise of them – get wide coverage in the medical press and it is not difficult for doctors to keep up to date. Claims by research workers must, however, be considered cautiously and reports read with guarded scepticism, for these reports are sometimes biassed and many claims have been later shown to be unfounded.

A cure for diabetes

If all the insulin-producing cells in the pancreas have been destroyed, some other source of insulin is required and, as we shall see, attention is being directed to methods of implantation of such cells. But if diabetes is in its early stages, prior to the destruction of the Islet cells, the question arises whether the process causing the destruction can be stopped.

The most hopeful advance, here, is the suggestion that in many cases, possibly in most, the process responsible for the damage to the Islets of Langerhans is an 'auto-immune' one. Auto-immune disease is common and may affect many parts of the body. Normally, the immune system, which protects us against infection and cancer, recognises our own internal cells as being of a special privileged class and respects them. In auto-immune disease there is a local break-down of this self-recognition. Recently there has been an increasing recognition that this may be the way in which the Islets are damaged and diabetes caused.

This evidence comes from various sources. One of the cell types of the immune system responsible for destroying 'foreign' cells is the 'T' lymphocyte and 'T' lymphocytes specific to pancreas cells have been found. Antibodies to Islet cells have also been found, indicating fairly clearly what is going on. But the most impressive evidence is that drugs which control immune reactions can actually stop the progress of the damage to the Islet cells, if used early enough. The first drug to be shown to have this effect was Cyclosporin, but because this drug acts to block immune processes as a whole there are obvious dangers in its use.

A new drug, Ciamexone, is said to suppress the early stages of the auto-immune process without suppressing resistance to infection or promoting growth of cancers. A report from West Germany, in the *Lancet* in September 1986, describes how eleven patients with newly diagnosed insulin-dependent diabetes agreed to treatment with Ciamexone. Of these, three were apparently cured and have required no insulin for a year so far; one patient, who appeared to be cured for three months, stopped taking the drug and returned to the diabetic state within two weeks. Four others showed a considerable improvement so that much lower doses of insulin were needed. The other three patients were not helped. In all, the drug was well tolerated and side effects were not a problem.

The drug was considered so promising that a large trial was set up in twenty centres in Germany, Switzerland and Austria to study 120 patients. The outcome is awaited with interest.

Transplants

Many diabetics, reading about kidney and heart–lung transplants, very naturally wonder why they can't have a pancreas transplant and be permanently cured. Unfortunately, the matter is not so simple. You must appreciate that major organ transplant surgery is done only in those cases where the alternatives are to leave the patient either to die or to suffer an intolerably poor quality of life. In these circumstances surgeons feel justified – and their patients agree with them – in taking major risks and in doing procedures which carry high mortality rates. Most people would gladly accept a 60 per cent chance of survival if the alternative is certain death within a few weeks or months.

To transplant an organ successfully, it is necessary to frustrate the body's natural defence mechanisms – which would otherwise immediately get to work on the transplanted organ and destroy it. The drugs which are used for this purpose – steroids and 'cytotoxic' agents – are very powerful and often have unpleasant side effects, and make the patient dangerously susceptible to infection and other hazards. So you will see that organ transplant is hardly justified in diabetes when the cure would almost certainly be worse than the disease. The additional susceptibility of the diabetic to infection is nothing compared to that of the transplant patient who has had to be 'immuno-compromised'.

Some pancreas transplants have been done, but these were in patients who were having kidney transplants for terminal diabetic nephropathy. Because these patients were, necessarily, very advanced diabetics with widespread complications, the results were not very good. If a well-controlled insulin-dependent diabetic had to have a heart or other transplant, it might be thought reasonable to do a pancreas transplant at the same time. But, on the other hand, the surgeon might well feel that the additional risk to the patient from, for instance, the release of pancreatic digestive enzyme, or from organ rejection, would be unjustified.

What about transplantation of the Islets of Langerhans, only? This seems to be a more realistic proposition and experiments have been encouraging. Islet cells have been implanted into the liver or spleen of diabetic animals and the cells have survived. In some cases these cells have responded to changes in the blood sugar by producing appropriate amounts of insulin, and some of the animals have actually been cured of their diabetes. There are, of course, problems. Islet cells from one individual are 'foreign' tissue to another and, unless prevented, rejection occurs. An exciting advance, in this area, is described below. The isolation of living Islet cells from the pancreas of human donors also presents major technical and ethical problems.

Research into immunology, which is one of the fastest-growing sectors of biological knowledge, together with the development of new and safer drugs for the control of rejection, is likely to lead to advances which will make transplantation safer and more feasible for a wider range of patients. It seems at least possible that Islet of Langerhans transplantation will succeed.

Microencapsulation

We have seen that the major problem with implanted Islet cells is that, because they are 'foreign', they are at once attacked by the immune system and destroyed. The weapons used by the immune system are fairly large proteins called antibodies and these are considerably larger than insulin molecules. So why not pack up the donor Islet of Langerhans cells in a porous bag with holes large enough to let the insulin out but too small to let the antibodies in?

This brilliant idea is, in fact, being following up right now and research is going on to produce tiny plastic spheres with exactly these properties. The idea, called micro-encapsulation, was developed and patented by a company called Damon Biotech and they are working, in conjunction with Canada's Connaught insulin laboratories, to perfect the method. So far it has not been tried in humans, but animal experiments have shown that an injection of these tiny Islet-containing spheres – they are small enough to be injected through an ordinary hypodermic needle – can successfully control diabetes for more than two years.

It seems that both the shape of the microcapsules and the placement of the Islet cells within them are important and it was proposed to prepare samples of these under weightless conditions in the space shuttle, in mid-1988. Tragically, the shuttle disaster is likely to delay this work.

Insulin by mouth

This, the dream of all insulin-dependent diabetics, has also been the subject of much research. I have already explained that insulin, being a protein, is digested and destroyed if eaten. But if insulin molecules are wrapped around with other substances, such as fats, they can be protected from digestion and may be absorbed intact. The trouble, so far, is that it has been found very difficult to ensure a predictable rate of absorption and release into the blood-stream. There are obviously many different ways in which insulin can be protected from digestion but most of these will also have an adverse effect on absorption. Research continues.

Insulin by inhalation

Recent experiments have shown that if insulin is combined with detergent-like substances, such as bile salts, and applied to the inside of the nose as an aerosol, sufficient quantities can be absorbed into the blood-stream to control the blood sugar levels in diabetics. There are, of course, problems, not the least being the difficulty of controlling the dosage, and it is not yet clear whether this idea is really feasible. It is, however, a most interesting line of research and development may lead to an important advance for insulin-dependent diabetics.

Pure insulin

Production of human insulin by 'recombinant DNA' genetic engineering is now well established. It is still expensive but promises to become, in the end, the cheapest and best way of obtaining medical insulin. The great advantage is that the insulin produced in this way is identical to human insulin and will not produce the antibodies commonly resulting from beef insulin and even from purified pork insulin. At present recombinant DNA-produced insulin is used largely for people with antibody problems, but we may expect, in the future, that it will be available to all insulin-dependent diabetics. This will be of special advantage to those 'brittle' diabetics requiring large doses (more than 100 units a day) for these often develop antibody problems which complicate control.

Better control of blood sugar

Blood sugar regulation by urine testing is indirect and rather crude. All diabetic specialists agree that it is much better, if possible, to check the blood sugar by direct measurement of the sugar in a blood specimen. In the past this has required laboratory facilities and the main disadvantage has been that, because of the time necessary to get the blood sample to the lab and because of queues in the laboratory and delays in completing report documentation, the result has always been retrospective. But with the development of individual personal monitors, such as the Glucochek meter, all this has changed, and you can now find out your blood sugar level, at any time. These meters work by measuring, with a remarkable degree of accuracy, the colour changes that occur with different glucose concentrations when a drop of blood is allowed to fall on a special strip. With the Ames 'Dextrostix' strip, a drop of blood is allowed to act for exactly 60 seconds (some meters have a timer) and is then washed off and blotted. The result can be read off at once.

It is quite certain that more, and cheaper, personal monitors will be developed and that blood sugar measurement, at home, will become commoner. This will be a major step forward in diabetic control and it is to be hoped that some far-sighted administrator, recognising the long-term savings that would result if, by this means, fewer diabetics developed complications, will authorise the issue of personal monitors on the NHS.

Continuous controlled infusion of insulin

The idea of this method is to try to mimic the normal situation by giving a continuous slow injection of insulin equivalent to the constant low output from the pancreas, and to deliver boosts in the dosage before each meal. The continuous flow of insulin is achieved by a special pump, which delivers carefully measured volumes of short-acting insulin, usually under the skin of the abdomen. In this method, the dosage is decided by estimation, and by experience, based on blood-sugar measurements.

But a much more sophisticated possibility, and one which has been successfully used under research conditions, is to convert this into a controlled 'feedback' system in which the dosage of insulin is automatically and constantly adjusted in accordance with 'real time' measurements of blood glucose. Such a method, based on continuous monitoring of blood sugar, required microcomputer control, but this is now a commonplace type of application.

Again, there are difficulties. The equipment is extremely expensive (the Biostator Controller developed in Indiana, cost $55,000 in 1982) and cannot easily be made light and compact enough to be convenient and portable. It will be some time before such equipment can be developed which does not severely restrict activity. The risks of breakdown or of the dislodging of the infusion needle, are considerable, and the constant presence of an opening in the skin leads to a tendency to infection. But the method is excellent in principle, and is capable of accurate control as has been shown by trials monitored by glycosylated haemoglobin levels and by the state of well-being of the patients taking part. The method, in its fully developed form, really amounts to the use of an 'artificial pancreas' and technological developments are likely to make it more practicable in the future.

GLOSSARY

Adrenaline A hormone from the adrenal glands which is released in times of stress and which mobilises sugar from the liver. It also causes some of the symptoms of hypoglycaemia.

Albustix A urine-testing strip which detects the presence of albumin. Albumin in the urine is almost always abnormal and suggests kidney disease.

Alpha cells The cells of the Islets of Langerhans which produce the anti-insulin hormone Glucagon. See *Beta cells*.

Amino acids These are the 'building bricks' of protein molecules. Digestion of protein in the bowel releases amino acids, which are absorbed into the blood-stream after a protein meal. Amino acids can also be released from muscles and used by the liver to manufacture new glucose (see *Gluconeogenesis*).

Angiopathy Disease of blood vessels. One of the principal complications of diabetes. Both large and small vessels are involved. See *Vascular disease*.

Antibodies Protein substances made by certain white cells in the blood ('lymphocytes') to combat 'foreign' invaders, such as germs or injected substances. Non-human insulin often stimulates antibody formation. Allergy is related to antibody action.

Atheroma A disease of large blood vessels (arteries) in which fatty material is deposited in the wall. Can lead to narrowing, and even total obstruction, by subsequent clotting of the blood.

Beta blockers A class of drugs used in the treatment of high blood pressure and heart disease. Their danger, to diabetics, is that they interfere with the action of adrenaline and so may reduce needed sugar production and cause hypoglycaemia. May also reduce awareness of hypoglycaemia by the absence of the adrenaline effects.

Beta cells The cells of the Islets of Langerhans, in the pancreas, which, in healthy people, produce insulin. In diabetes, these cells produce less, or no, insulin.

Blood sugar It is essential for brain survival and normal health that the blood should contain a minimum amount of glucose at all times. A drop below this level is called 'hypoglycaemia' and a rise above the level at which glucose 'spills' over into the urine is called 'hyperglycaemia'. The latter is a feature of diabetes.

Blood sugar monitoring The direct measuring of the blood glucose levels. A most important advance in the management of diabetes. Should be more widespread.

Brittle diabetes Diabetes which goes easily out of control. Sometimes thought to be a characteristic of the particular patient's illness, but is usually the result of poor cooperation with diet or insulin dosage.

Caesarian section The surgical removal of the unborn child through an abdominal incision. Often done to save the child of a diabetic mother.

Carbohydrate One of the three main constituents of food (the others being protein and fat) and the largest source of calories in most diets. All sugars, starches and cellulose are carbohydrates. Bread, potatoes, pasta, cakes and biscuits are mainly carbohydrate. Diabetics should take at least half of their calories in the form of carbohydrate, but should concentrate on the 'slow-release' form (see Ch. 6).

Cataract Opacification of the internal lenses of the eyes. Very common in older people and tends to occur at a rather earlier age in diabetics. A sudden-onset form of cataract may occur in young diabetics, but this is very rare.

Clinistix One of the popular forms of sugar-detection test. Very sensitive. The strip is dipped in urine and the colour change read in 10 seconds. Will detect the smallest traces of glucose.

Clinitest This is a 'quantitative' urine test for sugar. Five drops of urine and ten drops of water are put in a test-tube and the Clinitest tablet added. The colour change shows sugar concentrations of from ¼ per cent to 2 per cent. May be unreliable if you are taking salicylates or certain antibiotics or if you are pregnant.

Continuous insulin infusion A recent method of diabetes management, designed to try to mimic the normal blood sugar levels.

Corticosteroids Steroids are produced by the adrenal glands in times of stress and act against insulin.

Dextrostix A strip, used in conjunction with a colour-measuring meter, such as the Glucochek, for testing blood glucose.

Diastix A urine-testing strip giving glucose percentages. Used to check diabetic control.

Enzyme A protein produced by living cells, which accelerates biochemical reactions. Most enzymes function within cells but some, such as the digestive enzyme of the pancreas, operate outside cells.

Fats One of the three chief ingredients of food. High calorie value – three times' that of carbohydrate, weight for weight. The body's chief long-term calorie store.

Fibre Dietary fibre is made of complex carbohydrate ('polysaccharides') and we do not have enzymes capable of digesting this. So fibre adds to the bulk of the food without increasing the calorie value. Good for the bowels. Fibrous foods release their carbohydrate slowly and minimise sudden undesirable rises in the blood sugar.

Gangrene Death of tissue, usually as a result of loss of the blood supply.

Glucagon   The 'Beta' cells of the Islets of Langerhans produce insulin. The 'Alpha' cells produce glucagon, which is a hormone that raises the blood sugar level by prompting release from liver glycogen and by gluconeogenesis. Thus it acts in the opposite way to insulin. Can be used, by injection, to treat hypoglycaemia.

Gluconeogenesis   Literally 'glucose new birth'. Gluconeogenesis is a vital mechanism that enables us to survive during periods of starvation. Glucose is manufactured by the liver from amino acids, using fats as fuel. The process occurs to an abnormal degree in diabetes and contributes to the high blood sugar levels. Associated, in diabetes, with the production of abnormal quantities of ketone bodies.

Glucose   The essential fuel of the body. Derived from carbohydrate in the diet and from amino acids, by gluconeogenesis. Is stored in the liver in the compact 'polyglucose' called glycogen.

Glucotest   A sensitive and reliable strip test for sugar in the urine. Dip in urine and read after 1 minute.

Glycogen   A polymer of glucose. Found in the liver and in muscles. The chief form of glucose storage in the body. Glucose is readily available, on demand, from glycogen. Both adrenaline and glucagon can prompt the release of glucose from glycogen.

Glycosuria   Sugar (glucose) in the urine. Does not normally occur, but is a feature of diabetes.

Glycosylated haemoglobin   Glucose combines with the haemoglobin in the red cells of the blood in proportion to the average blood sugar level during the previous life of the red cell. So a check of the glycosylated haemoglobin level gives a useful indication of whether the blood sugar levels have been high in the previous two months or so. It thus provides a check of the standard of diabetic control.

Hormone   A chemical substance produced in one part of the body which is then carried, by the blood, to another part where it exerts an important effect. The production of hormones is often regulated by feedback of information about the magnitude of the effect. Thus, insulin alters the blood sugar levels and the changes in these levels controls the output of insulin.

Hydramnios An excessive increase in the amount of the uterine fluid surrounding the foetus during pregnancy. Commoner in diabetics than in others.

Hyperglycaemia Excess sugar (glucose) in the blood. This is the hallmark of diabetes. Causes sugar to appear in the urine.

Hypoglycaemia Abnormally low levels of blood sugar. One of the main dangers in insulin-treated diabetes. Every diabetic should be familiar with the symptoms. May even occur during sleep. The treatment, which is urgent, is to take sugar.

Insulin The hormone chiefly responsible for controlling the amount and fate of the body glucose. It controls entry of glucose to all body tissues, especially to muscles and fat deposits. Secreted by the Beta cells of the Islets of Langerhans in the pancreas. Absence, or relative deficiency, of insulin causes diabetes.

Insulin dosage Dosage is in units. Formerly insulin was provided in three strengths – 20 units per ml, 40 units per ml and 80 units per ml. This sometimes caused difficulty with the interpretation of syringe markings. Insulin of strength 100 units per ml is now becoming standard.

Insulin-dependent diabetics Diabetics whose natural insulin production has been damaged or eliminated by disease. Unless given insulin by injection, such people will die.

Islets of Langerhans The insulin (Beta cells) and glucagon-producing (Alpha cells) tissues of the pancreas. Named after Paul Langerhans, who first described the small islands of cells scattered amongst the digestive enzyme-producing glandular tissue.

Ketodiastix A strip test for both sugar and ketone bodies in the urine.

Ketone bodies Acidic substances produced in abnormal quantity as a result of diabetic gyuconeogenesis. Breath smells fruity ('pear drops'). Ketosis can change the acidity of the blood and lead to coma and death.

Ketostix A test for ketones in the urine. Dip and read after 15 seconds.

Maturity-onset diabetes Diabetes starting relatively late in life. Insulin is still being produced, but in insufficient quantities relative to the need. Sometimes, this form of diabetes can be cured simply by dieting; often oral hypoglycaemic drugs are needed; occasionally, insulin. Sometimes called 'type 2' diabetes.

Nephropathy Disease of the kidney. One of the most serious complications of diabetes. Diabetic nephropathy results from damage both to small blood vessels and to the kidney structure itself.

Neuropathy Disorder of nerve tissue in which conduction is affected. Another diabetic complication. The result is loss of sensation, weakness or paralysis of muscles and other loss of function. May cause organic impotence.

Oedema Swelling of tissue due to accumulation of fluid within or under it. Tends to occur in dependent parts of the body. May be a sign of kidney or heart disease. Pressure of the finger on an area of oedematous skin will leave a temporary 'pit' which then slowly fills.

Pancreas The dual-function organ which manufactures protein-digesting enzymes but also the hormone insulin. Lies high in the abdomen, behind the stomach.

Pancreatic enzyme In response to a meal containing protein, this digestive juice is secreted and passed along the pancreatic duct into the small intestine. The enzyme breaks down protein to amino acids, which are then absorbed into the blood-stream.

Protein   Meat. The main constituent of muscle. An important and essential element in the diet. Made of amino acids. The liver can synthesise glucose from broken-down protein.

Pyelonephritis   An infection of the kidney and of the urine-collecting system connected to it. Because of the tendency to infection in diabetes, patients with diabetic nephropathy may develop pyelonephritis.

Recombinant DNA   A part of the genetic blueprint, taken from one individual and inserted into another living cell, such as a bacterium, as a result of which the recipient cell manufactures a new protein, such as insulin. This is now an established way of manufacturing human insulin for medicinal purposes.

Renal threshold   The level of blood sugar at which the kidney allows sugar to appear in the urine. Sugar in the urine is usually a sign of diabetes, indicating that the blood sugar level is too high, but it may be due to a low renal threshold. This is common in pregnancy. The normal renal threshold is around 10 millimoles per litre.

Retinopathy   A disorder of the retina arising from damage to small blood vessels. One of the main complications of diabetes. Severe diabetic retinopathy is the commonest cause of blindness in middle age, but it can be effectively treated. Diabetics should be checked regularly – about once a year – for retinopathy.

Sugar   A carbohydrate. In the context of diabetes, 'sugar' means 'glucose'.

Sulphonylureas   The most important group of drugs used, in the form of tablets, for the treatment of maturity-onset diabetes. Oral hypoglycaemic agents.

Thrombosis   The clotting of blood within a blood vessel so that the flow is obstructed. Often caused by atheroma. Coronary thrombosis is an example.

Thrush   An infection with the fungus *Candida albicans*. Common in diabetes, especially in moist, dark areas. Effective treatments exist.

Toxaemia of pregnancy   A triad of signs – high blood pressure, albumin in the urine and oedema – which give warning of the risk of the serious convulsive disorder of 'eclampsia'. More common in diabetics than in others. Should always be detected by good ante-natal surveillance. If necessary, pregnancy may have to be terminated.

Trichophyton   A fungus which infects skin causing 'athletes' foot', 'crutch rot', 'ringworm', etc. Diabetics are more prone than others. Treatment is not difficult.

Vascular disease   Disease of blood vessels, mainly arteries. Both large and small vessels are affected in diabetes, with different consequences. 'Microvascular disease' (very small vessels) causes retinopathy, nephropathy and neuropathy, while 'macrovascular disease' causes 'atheroma' and the risk of major shut-down in blood supply. Effects such as coronary thrombosis or gangrene of extremities may result.

INDEX

120

121

RECIPES FOR DIABETICS:
by Billie Little and Penny Thorup

A DIABETIC DIET DOESN'T HAVE TO BE DULL!

When diabetes is diagnosed, a doctor usually gives the patient a list of foods to eat, in what quantity and at what intervals. Because standard cookbooks rarely supply the information needed to calculate a diabetic's individual requirements, many patients rely solely on a few drab, but safe, tested and measured dishes – a diet of unremitting monotony.

This book will change that. RECIPES FOR DIABETICS offers taste-tested marvellous main dishes, exotic and easy sauces, lively desserts, lip-smacking snacks, menu plans and much more.

Plus the simple but essential nutritive charts lacking in other cookbooks to guide you in preparing attractive, unusual, satisfying and varied meals that conform to the individual dietetic needs of the diabetic – and that are flavourful enough to satisfy the non-diabetic as well.

0 553 17274 3   £3.95

HOMEOPATHIC MEDICINE AT HOME
by Maesimund B. Panos M.D. and Jane Heimlich

Alternative Medicine the natural way in your own home

HOW TO CHOOSE AND USE HOMEOPATHIC TREATMENT

Homeopathy has long been recognised as an effective alternative to modern medical techniques, with the bonus that homeopathic remedies are non-toxic, safe for children and pregnant women and do not cause side-effects.

HOMEOPATHIC MEDICINE AT HOME is a comprehensive and practical guide to self-help homeopathy and tells you how to treat minor ailments, deal with emergencies and how to prescribe for yourself and your family.

- Your Home Remedy Kit
- What to do for Accidents
- A Happier Baby with Homeopathic Care
- How to Prevent and Treat Colds, Coughs, Ear-ache, Indigestion
- Your Growing Child
- What Homeopathy can do for Women
- Keeping your Pets Healthy

0 552 99244 5 &4.95

THE PATIENT'S COMPANION
by Dr. Vernon Coleman

'Definitely a worthwhile buy'
Woman's Own

'. . . a useful reference tool for the medicine cupboard'
The Times

'A mine of highly readable, well-organised information'
Company

The Patient's Companion was first published as *The Good Medicine Guide*, and has now been completely revised and updated for this new paperback edition.

Dr. Vernon Coleman is one of Britain's bestselling writers on medicine and this excellent reference book has been written to help everyone to get the very best health care for themselves and their families.

* how to read a prescription
* what to stock in your medicine cupboard
* what to do when someone dies
* what to take to hospital
* what a form FP 95 is (and 35 other forms that doctors hand out to patients)
* how to leave your body to a medical school
* how to change your doctor
* how to seek advice when going abroad
* what vaccinations you and your child need

0 552 12734 5   £3.95

NEW WAYS TO LOWER YOUR BLOOD PRESSURE
by Claire Safran

Learn How To Control Your High Blood Pressure

High Blood Pressure, or Hypertension, is widely recognised as one of the major risk factors in causing heart disease or strokes.

NEW WAYS TO LOWER YOUR BLOOD PRESSURE by award-winning writer Claire Safran will tell you everything your doctor may not have time for and sorts out current research, new ideas, approaches and treatments in a clear, easy-to-follow style.

Should you or shouldn't you cut out salt? What about your diet? What about the different drugs? Will meditation help you? Today there are more answers and more choices open to you than ever before. Claire Safran has information on what the best doctors say, and examines the range of treatments and the full repertory of cures and remedies. Let this valuable book help you choose the ways that will work for you. The more ideas you try, the quicker your blood pressure will come down and the healthier you'll be.

* New approaches to exercise
* New ways of looking at your diet
* New ideas about salt
* Most self-help methods will work within thirty days
* Includes a diet plan and recipes
* New healthy ways to reduce stress
* New relaxation techniques

0 552 12822 8 £3.50

NON FICTION AVAILABLE FROM PATHWAY

The prices shown below were correct at the time of going to press. However Transworld Publishers reserve the right to show new retail prices on covers which may differ from those previously advertised in the text or elsewhere.

ORDER FORM

All these books are available at your book shop or newsagent, or can be ordered direct from the publisher. Just tick the titles you want and fill in the form below.

Transworld Publishers, Cash Sales Department,
61-63 Uxbridge Road, Ealing, London, W5 5SA

Please send cheque or postal order, not cash. All cheques and postal orders must be in £ sterling and made payable to Transworld Publishers Ltd.

Please allow cost of book(s) plus the following for postage and packing:

U.K./Republic of Ireland Customers:
Orders in excess of £5; no charge
Orders under £5; add 50p

Overseas Customers:
All orders; add £1.50

NAME (Block Letters) . . . .

ADDRESS . . . .

. . . .